SMOOTHIES FOR WEIGHT GAIN

"Nourishing Recipes for a Healthier You"

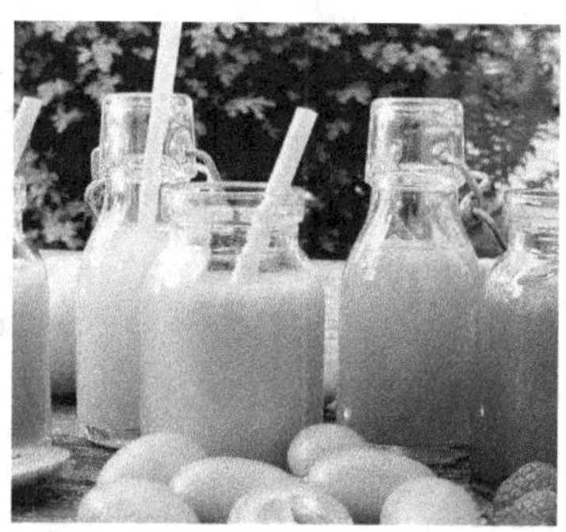

STEPHANIE C. JONES

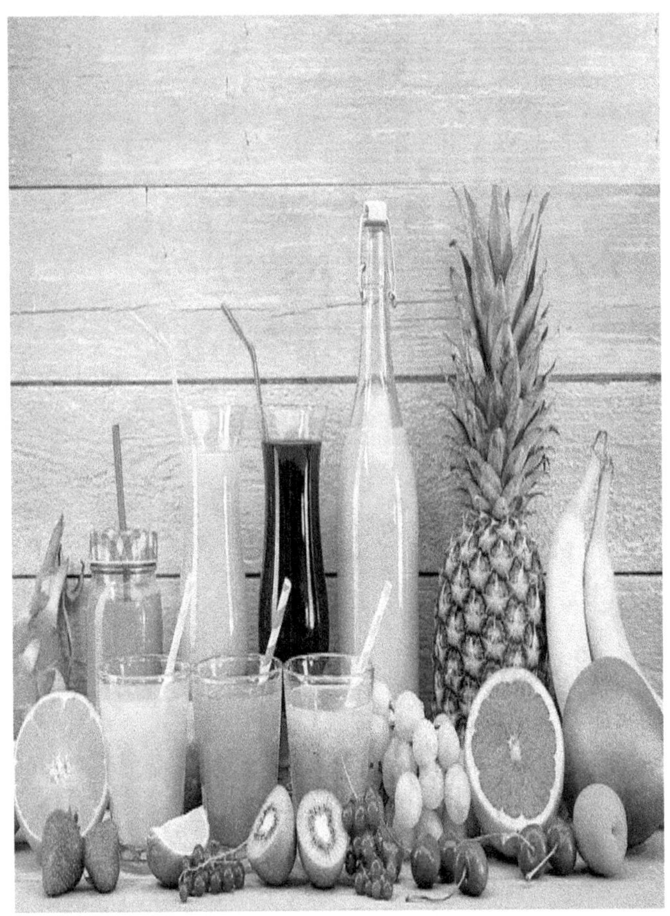

TABLE OF CONTENT

INTRODUCTION

- HOW TO USE THIS BOOK
- WHY SMOOTHIES ARE A GREAT WAY TO GAIN WEIGHT

CHAPTER 1

BUILDING THE PERFECT SMOOTHIE FOR WEIGHT GAIN

- THE KEY INGREDIENTS FOR WEIGHT GAIN SMOOTHIES
- TIPS FOR MAKING YOUR SMOOTHIES TASTE GREAT

CHAPTER 2

FRUIT-BASED SMOOTHIES

- BANANA AND PEANUT BUTTER SMOOTHIE
- BLUEBERRY AND YOGURT SMOOTHIE
- MANGO AND COCONUT MILK SMOOTHIE

CHAPTER 3

VEGETABLE-BASED SMOOTHIES

- ❖ SPINACH AND PEANUT BUTTER SMOOTHIE
- ❖ KALE AND BANANA SMOOTHIE
- ❖ CARROT AND GINGER SMOOTHIE
- ❖ BEET AND BERRY SMOOTHIE

CHAPTER 4

HIGH-CALORIE SMOOTHIES

- ❖ OATMEAL AND BANANA SMOOTHIE
- ❖ ALMOND BUTTER AND DATE SMOOTHIE
- ❖ AVOCADO AND CHOCOLATE SMOOTHIE

CHAPTER 5

PROTEIN-PACKED SMOOTHIES

- ❖ TOFU AND PEANUT BUTTER SMOOTHIE
- ❖ CHICKPEA AND BANANA SMOOTHIE
- ❖ QUINOA AND ALMOND MILK SMOOTHIE

CHAPTER 6

SUPERFOOD SMOOTHIES

- ❖ CHIA SEED AND BERRY SMOOTHIE
- ❖ MATCHA AND BANANA SMOOTHIE
- ❖ SPIRULINA AND MANGO SMOOTHIE
- ❖ MACA AND CHOCOLATE SMOOTHIE

CHAPTER 7

NUTRIENT-DENSE SMOOTHIES

- ❖ BROCCOLI AND PINEAPPLE SMOOTHIE
- ❖ PUMPKIN AND CINNAMON SMOOTHIE
- ❖ ZUCCHINI AND BANANA SMOOTHIE

CHAPTER 8

SMOOTHIES FOR BUILDING MUSCLE

- ❖ WHEY PROTEIN AND BANANA SMOOTHIE
- ❖ CREATINE AND BLUEBERRY SMOOTHIE

❖ BCAA AND MANGO SMOOTHIE

CHAPTER 9

SMOOTHIES FOR RECOVERY

❖ TURMERIC AND GINGER SMOOTHIE

❖ PINEAPPLE AND CUCUMBER SMOOTHIE

❖ STRAWBERRY AND ALMOND MILK SMOOTHIE

CHAPTER 10

SMOOTHIES FOR MEAL REPLACEMENT

❖ BERRY AND GREEK YOGURT MEAL REPLACEMENT SMOOTHIE.

❖ VANILLA AND BANANA MEAL REPLACEMENT SMOOTHIE.

❖ GREEN MEAL REPLACEMENT SMOOTHIE.

CHAPTER 11

SMOOTHIES FOR SPECIFIC DIETARY NEEDS

❖ GLUTEN-FREE SMOOTHIES

❖ DAIRY-FREE SMOOTHIES

❖ VEGAN SMOOTHIES

❖ LOW-SUGAR SMOOTHIES

CHAPTER 12

SMOOTHIES FOR BREAKFAST

❖ PEANUT BUTTER AND BANANA SMOOTHIE

❖ COFFEE AND CHOCOLATE SMOOTHIE

❖ MANGO AND COCONUT SMOOTHIE

CHAPTER 13

SMOOTHIES FOR SNACKS

❖ CINNAMON AND APPLE SMOOTHIE

❖ PEANUT BUTTER AND JELLY SMOOTHIE

❖ CHOCOLATE AND CHERRY SMOOTHIE

❖ RASPBERRY AND ALMOND MILK SMOOTHIE

CHAPTER 14

SMOOTHIES FOR DESSERT

❖ KEY LIME PIE SMOOTHIE

❖ STRAWBERRY CHEESECAKE SMOOTHIE

* <u>BANANA BREAD SMOOTHIE</u>

<u>CHAPTER 15</u>

<u>SMOOTHIES FOR KIDS</u>

* <u>BANANA AND NUTELLA SMOOTHIE</u>
* <u>STRAWBERRY AND VANILLA YOGURT SMOOTHIE</u>
* <u>ORANGE AND CARROT SMOOTHIE</u>
* <u>PEANUT BUTTER AND JELLY SMOOTHIE</u>

<u>CHAPTER 16</u>

<u>SMOOTHIES FOR SPECIAL OCCASIONS</u>

* <u>CHRISTMAS SMOOTHIE</u>
* <u>HALLOWEEN SMOOTHIE</u>
* <u>VALENTINE'S DAY SMOOTHIE</u>

<u>RECIPES TIMETABLE</u>

INTRODUCTION

If you're looking to gain weight in a healthy and delicious way, then you've come to the right place! **"The Smoothies for Weight Gain book"** is your ultimate guide to creating nutritious and tasty smoothies that will help you pack on the pounds.

While many people focus on losing weight, gaining weight can be just as challenging, especially for those who struggle to consume enough calories. Smoothies are an easy and convenient way to increase your calorie intake while also providing your body with essential nutrients.

In this book, you'll find a variety of smoothie recipes that are specifically designed to help you gain weight. These recipes are made with wholesome, nutrient-dense ingredients that will provide your body with the fuel it needs to build muscle and increase your overall mass.

We will also be focusing on smoothie recipes that are not only delicious but also packed with essential vitamins and minerals that your body needs to function at its best. We'll also provide tips on how to customize each recipe to meet your individual needs and preferences.

So whether you're looking for a quick breakfast option, a post-workout snack, or a refreshing afternoon treat, this book has got you covered. With a variety of flavors and ingredients to choose from, you're sure to find a smoothie recipe that fits your taste buds and supports your weight gain goals.

So let's get blending and start on your journey to healthy weight gain!

HOW TO USE THIS BOOK

Choose the right ingredients: Look for smoothie recipes that use ingredients that are high in calories and healthy fats such as bananas, avocado, nut butter, coconut milk, and Greek yogurt.

Measure ingredients properly: Be sure to measure your ingredients accurately to ensure that you are getting the right amount of nutrients and calories from each smoothie.

Experiment with different recipes: Try different recipes from the book to find the ones that taste the best to you and provide the most benefits in terms of weight gain.

Incorporate smoothies into your diet: Drink a smoothie as a snack or as a meal replacement to help you consume more calories throughout the day.

Track your progress: Keep track of your weight and how you feel after incorporating smoothies into your diet. This will help you determine if they are helping you achieve your weight gain goals.

Customize the recipes: You can also customize the recipes to fit your personal preferences or dietary needs. For example, if you are lactose intolerant, you can substitute dairy milk with almond milk or coconut milk.

Consider adding supplements: You can also consider adding supplements to your smoothies, such as protein powder or weight gain powder, to help you reach your calorie and nutrient goals.

Use a blender: Use a blender to mix your ingredients thoroughly and achieve a smooth texture. A high-powered blender is recommended for blending tougher ingredients like frozen fruits and vegetables.

Drink your smoothie immediately: It's best to drink your smoothie immediately after making it to ensure that you are getting the maximum amount of nutrients from the ingredients.

Balance your diet: While smoothies can be a great way to gain weight, it's important to balance your diet with other healthy foods such as lean protein, whole grains, and vegetables.

Be patient: Gaining weight takes time, so be patient and consistent with your smoothie intake and your overall diet and exercise routine.

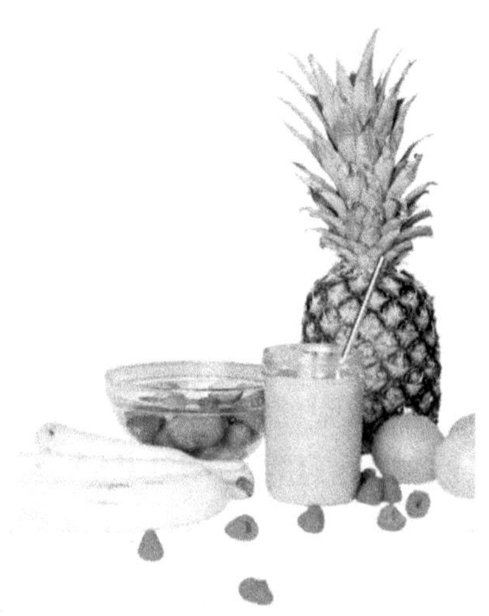

WHY SMOOTHIES ARE A GREAT WAY TO GAIN WEIGHT

Smoothies may have a high calorie content, particularly if you include calorie-dense foods like nut butters, avocado, and coconut milk. A calorie surplus, which may result in weight gain, is produced when you consume more calories than your body burns each day.

Smoothies are nutrient-dense and a fantastic method to get the nutrients your body needs to gain weight. You may include foods high in vitamins and minerals, such as fruits and vegetables, as well as foods high in protein, such as milk, yogurt, or protein powders, which is crucial for gaining muscle growth.

Smoothies are simple to digest, which allows for efficient absorption of the nutrients by the body. You want to maximize the quantity of nutrients your body can absorb, so this is particularly crucial if you're attempting to gain weight.

Smoothies may be greatly customized, and the ingredients can be changed to suit your own requirements. For instance, if your goal is to gain weight or develop muscle, you might increase your protein intake or your intake of good fats.

Smoothies are a practical alternative for those with hectic schedules since they are fast and simple to make. Smoothies are simple to prepare and take just a few minutes, so you can quickly include them to your regular routine.

Smoothies are an excellent method to boost your appetite if you are having trouble eating enough meals. Prior to a meal, consuming a smoothie might aid to enhance appetite and make it simpler to ingest more calories.

Variety of tastes: Smoothies come in a wide range of tastes, so you may choose a recipe that you like and are eager to consume. This may make it simpler for you to include smoothies in your diet on a regular basis.

Smoothies may be consumed while on the go, making them a fantastic alternative for folks who are always on the go. Pour your smoothie into a travel cup and take it to work or school with you.

Smoothies may also help you stay hydrated, which is vital for your general health and wellness. Many smoothie recipes call for water-rich fruits and vegetables, which may help you stay hydrated throughout the day.

Cost-Effective: Making your own smoothies at home with items you already own will help you gain weight without breaking the bank. The cost of pricey meal replacement drinks or weight gain supplements may be reduced as a result.

Smoothies are a terrific method to enhance digestion, which is crucial for general health and well-being. Leafy greens, fruit that is high in fiber, and probiotics are all components that are often included in smoothie recipes because they may aid with digestion and encourage regular bowel movements.

Smoothies may be an excellent approach to help muscle repair after exercise. Protein may aid in repairing muscle tissue and preventing muscular breakdown, which is crucial for gaining muscle growth.

Smoothies are a fantastic approach to help regulate blood sugar levels, particularly if you already have diabetes or are at risk of acquiring it. By including components like high-fiber fruits, protein, and good fats, you may lessen the rate at which sugar enters your system and avoid blood sugar rises.

Smoothies may help with mental clarity, which is crucial for productivity and general well-being. Smoothies can also help with attention. Blueberries are a common addition in smoothie recipes because of their high antioxidant content, which may assist to prevent brain cell deterioration.

boost for the immune system: Smoothies are a fantastic method to boost the immune system, which is crucial for fending off sickness and disease. The immune system may be strengthened and general health can be improved by including substances like citrus fruits, ginger, and turmeric.

Smoothies are a terrific method to keep your weight in check, particularly if you have trouble with overeating or portion management. Smoothie consumption may help people manage their weight by reducing hunger and preventing overeating.

CHAPTER 1

BUILDING THE PERFECT SMOOTHIE FOR WEIGHT GAIN

THE KEY INGREDIENTS FOR WEIGHT GAIN SMOOTHIES

Protein Powder: Increasing your protein consumption, which is necessary for muscle development and repair, may be accomplished by including protein powder into your smoothie.

Nut Butter: Nut butter, such as peanut, almond, or cashew butter, boosts the nutritional value, protein, and calorie content of your smoothie.

Fruits: Fruits may provide critical vitamins and minerals as well as carbs for energy to your smoothie. Great choices include mangoes, berries, and bananas.

veggies: Including veggies like spinach, kale, or avocado in your smoothie may provide vital nutrients, fiber, and healthy fats.

Milk or Yogurt: Milk or yogurt may boost your smoothie's calories, protein, and calcium content.

Oats: Oats are a good source of fiber, carbs, and other essential elements for smoothies.

Sweeteners: You may include stevia, honey, or maple syrup to make your smoothie sweeter. Use of these should be moderated, however.

Ice: Including ice in your smoothie can help it become thicker and more refreshing.

It's crucial to remember that smoothies for weight growth should be drunk sparingly, along with a healthy diet and consistent exercise.

Greek yogurt is a fantastic source of protein, calcium, and probiotics, which may benefit your digestive system.

Cottage Cheese: Cottage cheese gives your smoothie a creamy texture and offers an excellent dose of calcium, minerals, and protein.

Chia Seeds: Chia seeds are rich in fiber and omega-3 fatty acids, two nutrients that might help you feel full.

Hemp Seeds: Hemp seeds are a great source of protein, good fats, and important vitamins and minerals including iron and magnesium.

Flaxseed: Flaxseed is an excellent source of omega-3 fatty acids and fiber, both of which may enhance heart health and facilitate digestion.

Coconut Oil: Coconut oil is an excellent source of beneficial fats that may boost energy and promote weight growth.

Nuts: Nuts like almonds, cashews, and walnuts may boost the protein, fiber, and healthy fat content of your smoothie.

Dates: Dates are a healthy sweetener that may also be a good source of fiber and potassium.

Cinnamon: Cinnamon may give your smoothie a sweet and spicy taste as well as significant antioxidant and anti-inflammatory properties.

Boosting energy, elevating mood, and enhancing libido are just a few of the benefits of the root vegetable maca powder.

Spirulina is an antioxidant- and protein-rich blue-green algae that is also high in other vital minerals.

Wheat germ is the most nutrient-dense component of the wheat kernel and an excellent source of fiber, vitamins, and minerals.

Silken Tofu: A vegan protein source, silken tofu may give your smoothie a creamy smoothness.

Avocado Oil: Rich in monounsaturated fatty acids, avocado oil may assist to strengthen the heart and encourage weight growth.

Dark Chocolate: In addition to adding a deep, chocolaty taste to your smoothie, dark chocolate also has valuable antioxidants and minerals.

MCT Oil: MCT oil is a kind of fat that the body can rapidly absorb. It may boost energy and assist with weight growth.

Bee Pollen: Bees produce a nutrient-rich material called pollen that contains essential vitamins, minerals, and amino acids.

As usual, it's important to utilize these products sparingly and balance them with a nutritious, well-balanced diet.

TIPS FOR MAKING YOUR SMOOTHIES TASTE GREAT

The most crucial element in creating a good smoothie is to use fresh, ripe fruit. To give your smoothie a naturally sweet flavor, make sure the fruit you choose is ripe and tasty.

Insert some liquid: For a creamy, smooth texture, use a liquid foundation for your smoothie, such as water, coconut water, milk, or a plant-based milk.

Combine flavors: Try out various fruit and vegetable combinations to see which taste combination suits you the best. To pack in more nutrients, think about adding some greens to your smoothie, such spinach or kale.

Enhance it with natural sweeteners: To give your smoothie a touch of sweetness, add natural sweeteners like honey, dates, or maple syrup.

Use frozen fruit: Using frozen fruit in place of fresh fruit will give your smoothie a creamier and thicker consistency. To have the same result, you may also add ice.

To make your smoothie more full and fulfilling, add additional protein in the form of nut butter or protein powder.

Don't forget the garnishes: To add some texture and taste to your smoothie, sprinkle some nuts, seeds, granola, or fresh fruit on top.

Use a high-speed blender: Your smoothies' texture and consistency might significantly change if you invest in a high-speed blender. Even the hardest components may be combined in a strong blender to create a smooth and creamy texture.

Spices like cinnamon, ginger, and nutmeg may give your smoothie some warmth and depth of taste. Find the spice combination you like most by experimenting with various spices.

Use frozen yogurt or ice cream: Using frozen yogurt or ice cream as a basis may give your drink a rich, creamy texture and make it more like a dessert than a smoothie.

Include some healthy fats: Healthy fats like avocado, nut butter, and coconut oil may increase the fullness and satisfaction of your smoothie. They may also give your beverage a richer, creamier flavor.

Superfoods like chia seeds, flaxseeds, and hemp seeds may give your smoothie a little more nutrition and texture. Additionally, they're a fantastic way to add fiber and some good fats to your beverage.

Use flavor-enhanced protein powder: If you want to add protein to your smoothie, flavor-enhanced protein powder may make your beverage taste wonderful. To get the right protein powder for your smoothie, consider its taste profile.

Add some citrus: Citrus fruits may give your smoothie some tang and freshness. Lemons and limes are two examples. Additionally, they might aid in bringing your drink's sweetness into balance.

Just keep in mind that there is no right or wrong method to create a smoothie. To identify the one you enjoy the best, you must experiment with various ingredients and taste pairings.

CHAPTER 2

FRUIT-BASED SMOOTHIES

BANANA AND PEANUT BUTTER SMOOTHIE

Banana and peanut butter smoothie is a great option for weight gain as it is packed with healthy fats, protein, and carbohydrates. Here's how to make a delicious and nutritious banana and peanut butter smoothie:

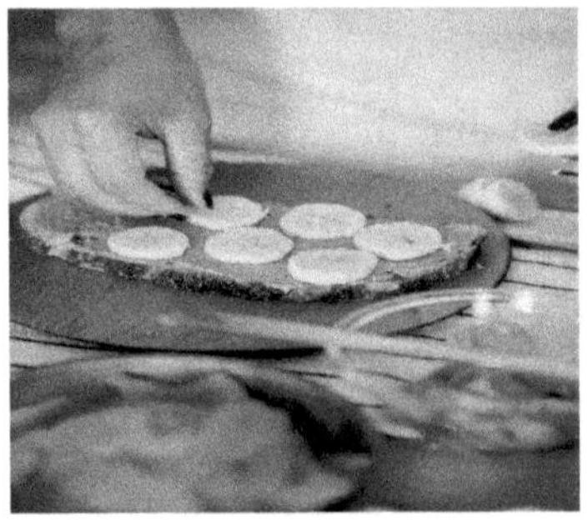

INGREDIENTS:

2 ripe bananas

2 tbsp peanut butter

1 cup milk (can use any milk of your choice)

1/2 cup Greek yogurt

1 tsp honey (optional)

1/4 tsp cinnamon (optional)

1/2 cup ice cubes

Instructions:

Begin by gathering all of your ingredients and preparing them for the smoothie.

Peel the bananas and chop them into small pieces.

Add the chopped bananas, peanut butter, Greek yogurt, milk, honey (if using), and cinnamon (if using) into a blender.

Blend the ingredients until smooth.

Add the ice cubes into the blender and continue blending until the smoothie is thick and creamy.

Pour the smoothie into a glass and enjoy!

TIPS:

If you want a thicker smoothie, use frozen bananas instead of fresh ones.

You can add more peanut butter if you prefer a stronger peanut butter taste.

Add more milk if the smoothie is too thick for your liking.

If you want to make the smoothie vegan, use a non-dairy milk and yogurt instead.

NUTRITIONAL INFORMATION (PER SERVING):

Calories: 428

Protein: 17g

Fat: 17g

Carbohydrates: 57g

Fiber: 5g

Sugar: 35g

Overall, the banana and peanut butter smoothie is a delicious and nutritious way to gain weight. It's packed with protein, healthy fats, and carbohydrates to help fuel your body and build muscle. Enjoy it as a snack or as part of your breakfast or post-workout routine.

BLUEBERRY AND YOGURT SMOOTHIE

Blueberry and Yogurt Smoothie is a delicious and nutritious way to gain weight. Here is a recipe to make a creamy and filling Blueberry and Yogurt Smoothie:

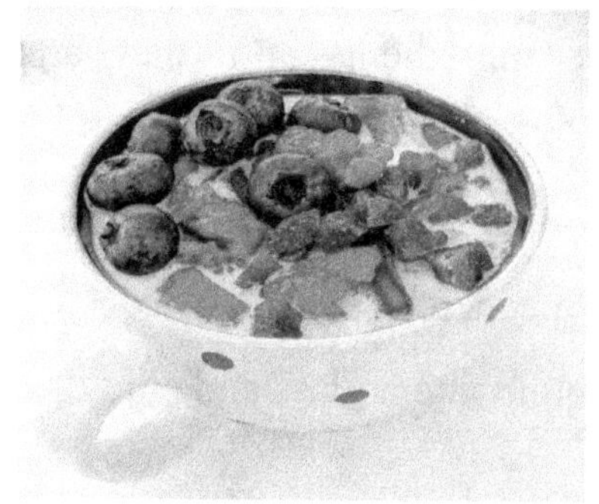

INGREDIENTS:

1 cup blueberries

1 cup plain yogurt

1 banana

1 tablespoon honey

1/4 cup oats

1 tablespoon almond butter

1 cup milk

INSTRUCTIONS:

Rinse the blueberries and set them aside.

Peel the banana and slice it into small pieces.

In a blender, add the blueberries, yogurt, banana, honey, oats, almond butter, and milk.

Blend all the ingredients until they are smooth and creamy.

Taste the smoothie and adjust the sweetness by adding more honey if needed.

Pour the smoothie into a glass and enjoy!

TIPS:

Use frozen blueberries to make the smoothie extra cold and thick.

Substitute the almond butter with peanut butter or any nut butter of your choice.

Use full-fat yogurt and milk for a creamier and more calorie-dense smoothie.

Add a scoop of vanilla protein powder to boost the protein content of the smoothie.

Top the smoothie with some granola or chopped nuts for some crunch

STRAWBERRY AND AVOCADO SMOOTHIE

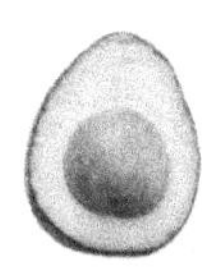

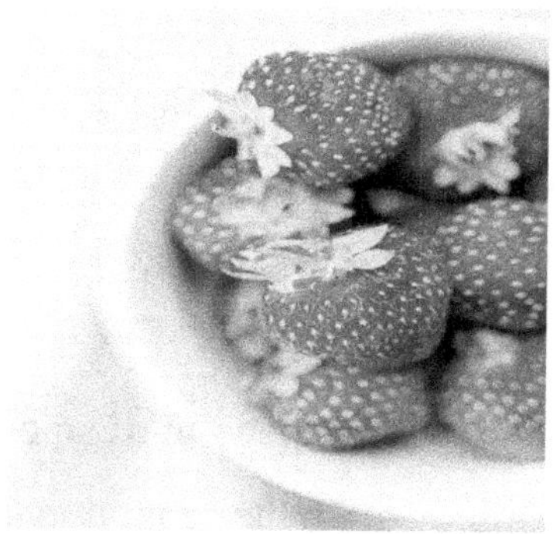

Here's a recipe for a delicious Strawberry and Avocado Smoothie that can help with weight gain:

INGREDIENTS:

1 cup fresh or frozen strawberries

1 ripe avocado

1 cup milk (dairy or non-dairy)

1/2 cup Greek yogurt

1 tbsp honey or maple syrup

1 tbsp chia seeds (optional)

1/2 tsp vanilla extract

INSTRUCTIONS:

Wash and hull the strawberries. Cut the avocado in half and remove the pit.

In a blender, combine the strawberries, avocado, milk, Greek yogurt, honey or maple syrup, chia seeds (if using), and vanilla extract.

Blend on high speed until smooth and creamy, for about 1-2 minutes. If the smoothie is too thick, you can add more milk or water to thin it out.
Pour the smoothie into a tall glass and enjoy immediately.

TIPS:

Use ripe avocados for the creamiest texture.
If you're using fresh strawberries, you can add a few ice cubes to make the smoothie more refreshing.
For an extra protein boost, you can add a scoop of protein powder or a tablespoon of peanut butter to the smoothie.

Store any leftover smoothie in an airtight container in the fridge for up to 24 hours. Shake well before serving.

Overall, this smoothie is a great way to add healthy calories and nutrients to your diet, thanks to the combination of protein-rich Greek yogurt, fiber-packed chia seeds, and healthy fats from avocado. Enjoy!

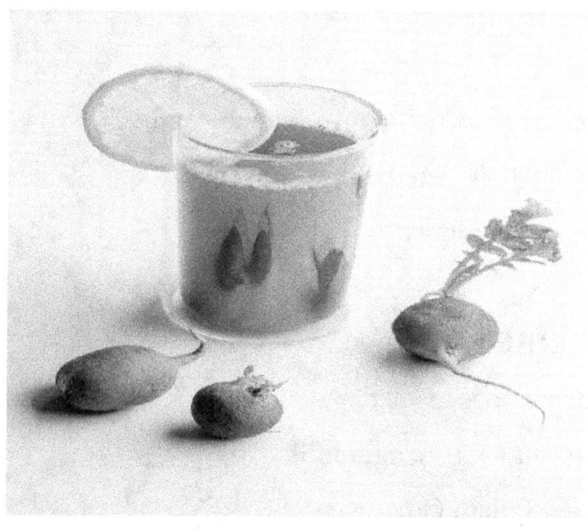

MANGO AND COCONUT MILK SMOOTHIE

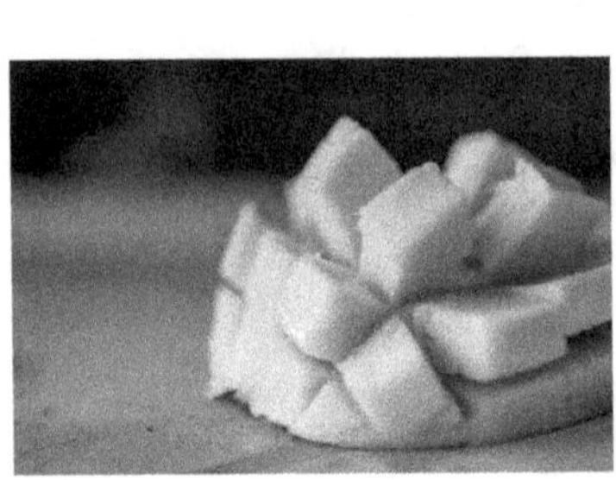 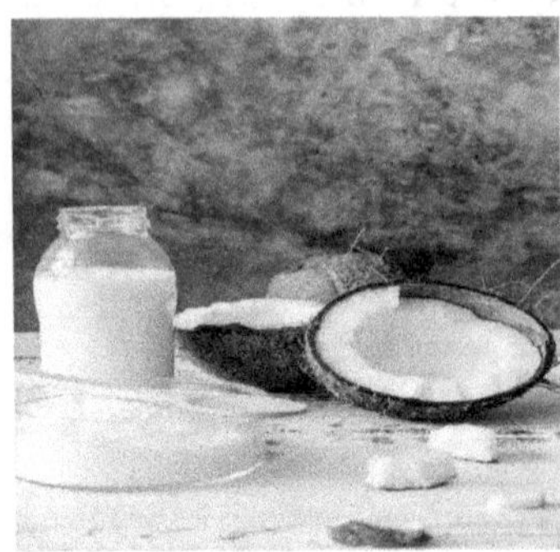

Recipe for a delicious Mango and Coconut Milk Smoothie that can help with weight gain. This recipe makes two servings.

INGREDIENTS:

2 ripe mangoes, peeled and chopped

1 can of full-fat coconut milk

1/2 cup of plain Greek yogurt

2 tablespoons of honey

1 teaspoon of vanilla extract

1/2 teaspoon of ground cinnamon

1/4 teaspoon of ground ginger

1/4 teaspoon of ground cardamom

1/4 teaspoon of sea salt

1 cup of ice cubes

INSTRUCTIONS:

Start by preparing your mangoes. Cut the flesh away from the pit and chop it into small pieces.

Add the chopped mangoes to your blender.

Open the can of coconut milk and add it to the blender.

Add the Greek yogurt, honey, vanilla extract, ground cinnamon, ground ginger, ground cardamom, and sea salt to the blender.

Add the ice cubes to the blender.

Blend all the ingredients together until smooth and creamy.

Taste the smoothie and adjust the sweetness to your liking by adding more honey if necessary.

Pour the smoothie into two glasses and serve immediately.

TIPS:

To make this smoothie even creamier, you can replace the Greek yogurt with coconut cream.

If you don't have fresh mangoes, you can use frozen mango chunks instead.

To increase the calorie content of this smoothie, you can add a tablespoon of almond butter or peanut butter to the blender.

You can also add a scoop of protein powder to the blender to make this smoothie more filling and satisfying.

Mangoes are high in fiber and vitamin C, while coconut milk is high in healthy fats and calories, making this smoothie a great choice for those looking to gain weight in a healthy way.

CHAPTER 3

VEGETABLE-BASED SMOOTHIES

SPINACH AND PEANUT BUTTER SMOOTHIE

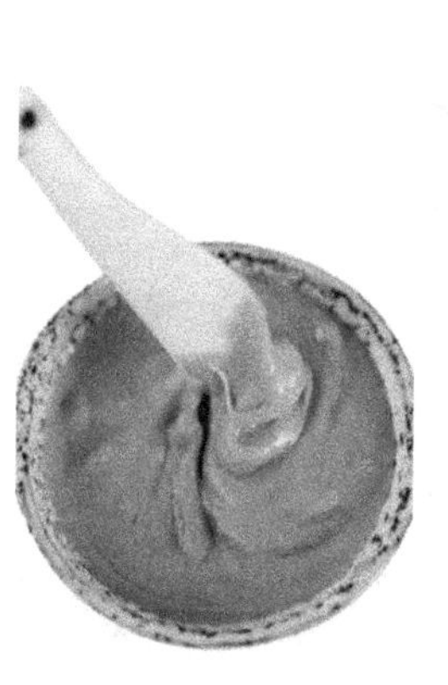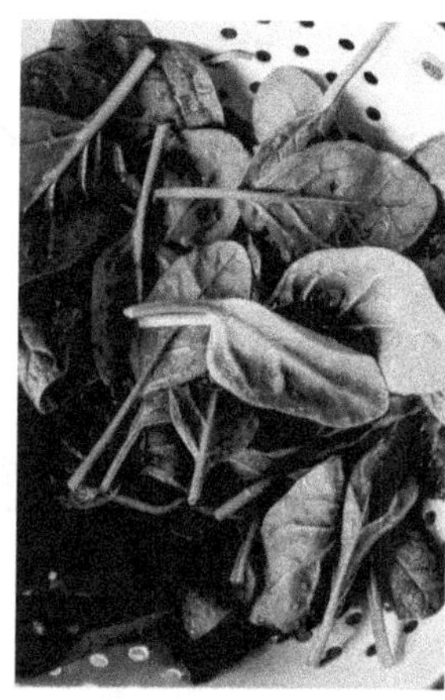

Spinach and peanut butter smoothie is a nutritious and delicious drink that can help you gain weight when combined with a balanced diet and exercise routine. Here is a step-by-step recipe to help you make your own spinach and peanut butter smoothie for weight gain:

INGREDIENTS:

2 cups fresh spinach leaves

1 ripe banana

1/4 cup peanut butter

1 cup unsweetened almond milk

1/2 cup plain Greek yogurt

1 tablespoon honey (optional)

1/2 teaspoon vanilla extract (optional)

1 scoop protein powder (optional)

INSTRUCTIONS:

Wash and prepare the spinach leaves. Remove any stems or tough pieces.

Cut the banana into small chunks.

Add the spinach leaves, banana, peanut butter, almond milk, and Greek yogurt into a blender.

If desired, add honey, vanilla extract, and protein powder to the blender as well.

Blend all the ingredients until they are well combined and smooth.

Pour the smoothie into a glass and enjoy immediately.

TIPS:

Use ripe bananas for a sweeter taste and smoother texture.

If you don't have almond milk, you can use any other type of milk, such as cow's milk or soy milk.

Greek yogurt adds protein and creaminess to the smoothie. If you are lactose intolerant, you can use a non-dairy yogurt instead.

If the smoothie is too thick, you can add more milk to thin it out. If it's too thin, you can add more banana or peanut butter to thicken it up.

To make the smoothie colder and more refreshing, you can add some ice cubes to the blender.

You can also add other ingredients to the smoothie to vary the flavor and nutrient content, such as berries, cocoa powder, chia seeds, or flax seeds.

Overall, spinach and peanut butter smoothie is a healthy and tasty way to gain weight and improve your nutrition. By following this recipe and customizing it to your preferences, you can create a delicious and satisfying drink that will help you achieve your weight gain goals.

KALE AND BANANA SMOOTHIE

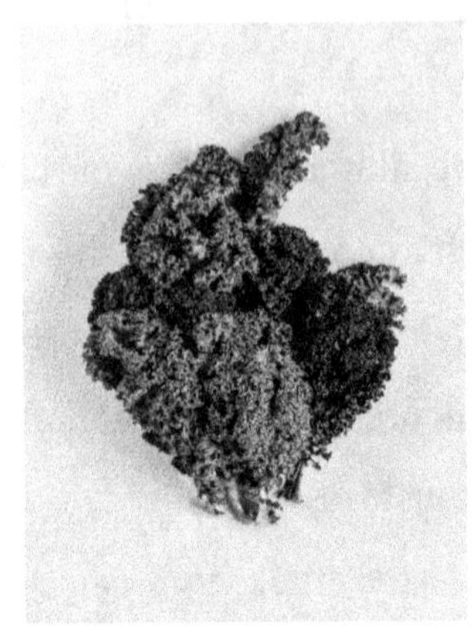

INGREDIENTS:

1 cup kale leaves, chopped

1 ripe banana

1/2 cup plain Greek yogurt

1/2 cup whole milk

1 tablespoon honey

1/4 teaspoon vanilla extract

1/4 teaspoon ground cinnamon

1/2 cup ice cubes

INSTRUCTIONS:

Wash the kale leaves thoroughly, and chop them into small pieces.

Peel the banana, and cut it into chunks.

Add the kale, banana, Greek yogurt, whole milk, honey, vanilla extract, and ground cinnamon to a blender.

Blend the ingredients until smooth and creamy.

Add the ice cubes to the blender, and blend again until the smoothie is thick and frothy.

Taste the smoothie, and adjust the sweetness or thickness as desired.

Pour the smoothie into a tall glass, and enjoy!

Kale is a nutrient-dense green vegetable that is low in calories but high in fiber, vitamins, and minerals. Bananas are a great source of carbohydrates, potassium, and natural sugars. Greek yogurt provides protein and probiotics, while whole milk adds extra calories and creaminess to the smoothie. Honey and vanilla extract add sweetness, while ground cinnamon adds a warm, spicy flavor. The ice cubes make the smoothie thick and frothy, and provide a refreshing chill.

To make this smoothie even more calorically dense, you can add a scoop of protein powder, a tablespoon of nut butter, or some avocado to the blender. You can also use a higher-fat milk, such as almond or coconut milk, instead of whole milk. Drink this smoothie as a snack or a meal replacement to help with weight gain. Enjoy!

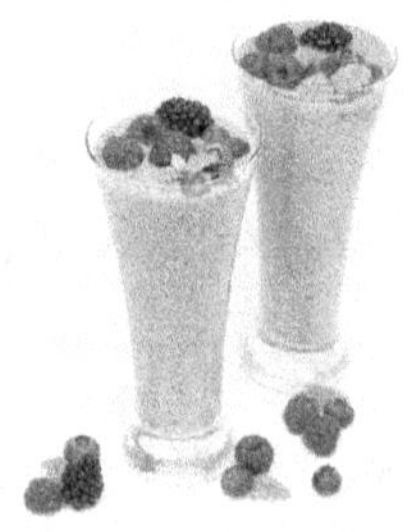

CARROT AND GINGER SMOOTHIE

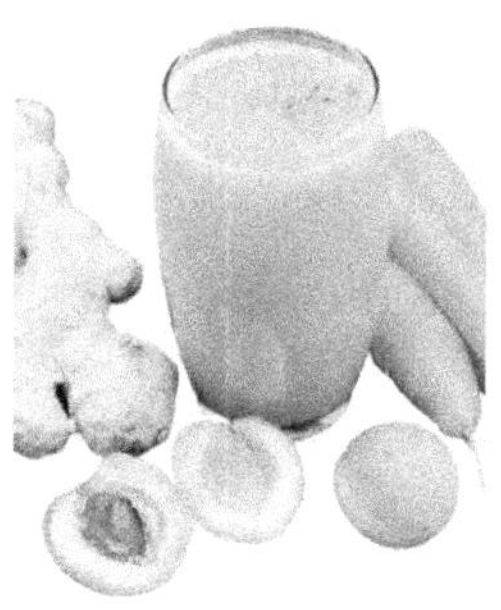

Carrot and Ginger smoothie is a delicious and healthy drink that can aid in weight gain. Here's a recipe for a long, satisfying drink:

INGREDIENTS:

2 medium-sized carrots, peeled and chopped

1-inch piece of fresh ginger, peeled and grated

1 ripe banana, peeled and chopped

1 cup of unsweetened almond milk (or any other plant-based milk)

1 tablespoon of honey or maple syrup (optional)

1 tablespoon of chia seeds (optional)

INSTRUCTIONS:

Wash, peel and chop the carrots into small pieces.

Grate the ginger and set it aside.

Peel the banana and chop it into small pieces.

Add the chopped carrots, grated ginger, and chopped banana to a blender.

Pour in the almond milk.

Blend on high speed until the mixture is smooth and creamy.

Taste the smoothie and add honey or maple syrup, if desired, for extra sweetness.

Add chia seeds, if desired, and blend for a few seconds until the seeds are well combined.

Pour the smoothie into a glass and serve immediately.

This smoothie is packed with nutrients that can aid in weight gain, such as protein, fiber, healthy fats, and vitamins. The chia seeds can also provide extra protein and fiber, making it a filling and satisfying drink. Enjoy!

BEET AND BERRY SMOOTHIE

Beet and berry smoothie is a nutritious and delicious way to gain weight. Here is a recipe for making a beet and berry smoothie:

INGREDIENTS:

1 medium-sized beetroot, peeled and chopped

1 cup mixed berries (such as strawberries, blueberries, and raspberries)

1 banana, peeled and sliced

1 cup milk (or dairy-free milk alternative)

1 tablespoon honey (optional)

1/2 teaspoon vanilla extract (optional)

INSTRUCTIONS:

Add the chopped beetroot and mixed berries to a blender.

Add the sliced banana, milk, honey, and vanilla extract (if using) to the blender.

Blend all the ingredients until smooth and creamy.

Taste the smoothie and adjust the sweetness if needed by adding more honey.

Pour the smoothie into a glass and serve chilled.

TIPS:

Use ripe bananas: Ripe bananas are sweeter and have a higher calorie count than unripe ones, making them an excellent addition to your smoothie.

Choose the right berries: Berries are low in calories, but they are also rich in vitamins, minerals, and antioxidants. Use a mix of different berries to get the maximum health benefits.

Use full-fat milk: Full-fat milk is high in calories and healthy fats, which can help you gain weight. If you are lactose intolerant or prefer a dairy-free alternative, you can use almond milk or coconut milk.

Add honey: Honey is a natural sweetener that can make your smoothie taste better. It is also a good source of carbohydrates, which can help you gain weight.

Add protein powder: If you want to increase your protein intake, you can add a scoop of protein powder to your smoothie. This will help you build muscle mass and gain weight.

Add healthy fats: Adding healthy fats like avocado, nuts, or nut butter can increase the calorie count of your smoothie and make it more filling.

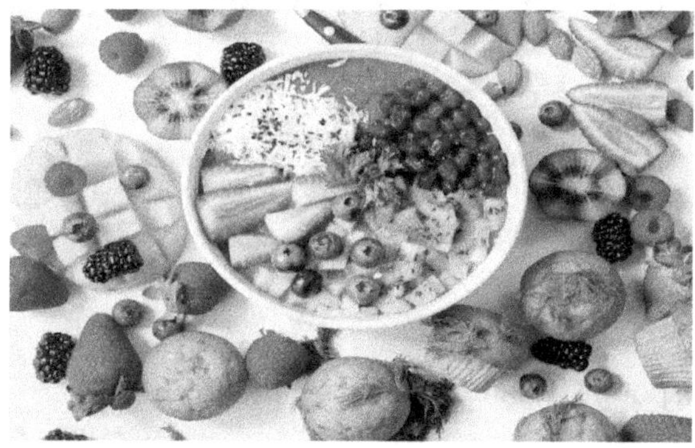

CHAPTER 4

HIGH-CALORIE SMOOTHIES

CHOCOLATE AND PEANUT BUTTER SMOOTHIE

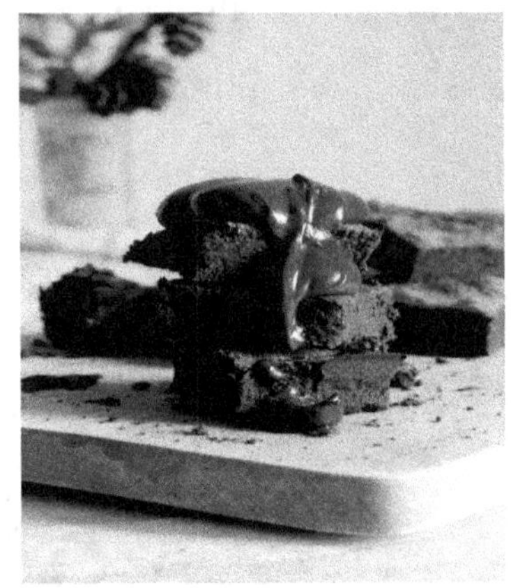

INGREDIENTS:

2 ripe bananas

2 tablespoons of natural peanut butter

1 tablespoon of unsweetened cocoa powder

1/2 cup of Greek yogurt

1/2 cup of whole milk

1 teaspoon of honey (optional)

1/2 teaspoon of vanilla extract

1 cup of ice cubes

INSTRUCTIONS:

Peel the bananas and slice them into small pieces.

Add the banana slices, peanut butter, cocoa powder, Greek yogurt, milk, honey (if using), and vanilla extract to a blender.

Add the ice cubes to the blender as well.

Blend all the ingredients until smooth and creamy.

Pour the smoothie into a glass and enjoy!

TIPS:

Use ripe bananas - they're sweeter and easier to blend than unripe bananas.

Use natural peanut butter that doesn't have added sugar or oils.

Use unsweetened cocoa powder to avoid adding unnecessary sugar to the smoothie.

Use Greek yogurt for added protein.

Use whole milk for extra calories and creaminess.

Use honey to add sweetness if needed, but keep in mind that it's an added sugar.

Add ice cubes to make the smoothie thicker and more refreshing.

Consider adding protein powder to the smoothie for extra calories and protein.

Drink the smoothie as a snack or meal replacement to help with weight gain.

Be mindful of portion sizes - while this smoothie can be helpful for weight gain, overeating can lead to unhealthy weight gain.

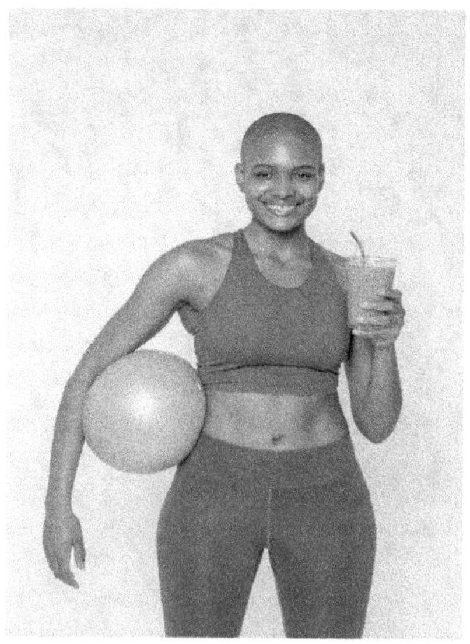

OATMEAL AND BANANA SMOOTHIE

INGREDIENTS:

1 cup of rolled oats

1 banana

1 cup of milk

1 tablespoon of honey

1/4 teaspoon of cinnamon

1/4 teaspoon of vanilla extract

1/2 cup of ice

INSTRUCTIONS:

Add rolled oats to a blender and pulse until they are finely ground.

Add the banana, milk, honey, cinnamon, vanilla extract, and ice to the blender with the ground oats.

Blend all ingredients until smooth and creamy.

Taste and adjust the sweetness with more honey, if needed.

Pour into a glass and enjoy!

TIPS:

Use whole milk instead of skim or low-fat milk to add more calories and healthy fats to the smoothie.

Add a scoop of protein powder to the smoothie for an extra protein boost that can aid in muscle growth and weight gain.

Use Greek yogurt instead of milk to add even more protein to the smoothie.

Try adding other fruits or veggies like spinach, berries, or avocado to increase the nutrient density of the smoothie without adding too many extra calories.

Consider adding a tablespoon of nut butter or coconut oil to the smoothie for some healthy fats and extra calories. Drink the smoothie as a snack or meal replacement to help with weight gain.

ALMOND BUTTER AND DATE SMOOTHIE

Almond Butter and Date Smoothie is a delicious and healthy way to gain weight. This smoothie is packed with nutrients and healthy fats that will help you reach your weight gain goals. Here is a recipe for almond butter and date smoothie along with some tips to make it more effective for weight gain.

INGREDIENTS:

2 ripe bananas

2 cups almond milk

2 tbsp almond butter

4 dates, pitted

1 tbsp honey

1 tsp vanilla extract

1/4 tsp cinnamon

1 scoop protein powder (optional)

INSTRUCTIONS:

Peel and slice the bananas and place them in a blender.

Add the almond milk, almond butter, dates, honey, vanilla extract, and cinnamon to the blender.

Blend all the ingredients until smooth and creamy.

Add a scoop of protein powder if desired and blend again.

Pour the smoothie into a glass and serve immediately.

TIPS:

Use full-fat ingredients: When making a smoothie for weight gain, it's important to use full-fat ingredients. Almond milk, almond butter, and dates are all rich in healthy fats that will help you gain weight in a healthy way.

Add protein powder: If you're trying to build muscle mass, adding a scoop of protein powder to your smoothie can help. Look for a protein powder that is low in sugar and high in protein.

Use ripe bananas: Ripe bananas are sweeter and easier to digest than unripe bananas. They also contain more nutrients, which is important when trying to gain weight.

Add oats: Adding oats to your smoothie can increase its calorie content and provide additional fiber and nutrients. Rolled oats are a great option because they blend well and don't add a lot of texture.

Customize to your taste: You can adjust the sweetness and thickness of your smoothie by adding more or less honey or almond milk. You can also add other ingredients like cocoa powder, chia seeds, or frozen fruit to customize the flavor.

Drink it after a workout: Drinking your smoothie after a workout can help your body absorb the nutrients more effectively and aid in muscle recovery and growth.

Pair it with a meal: Drinking a smoothie as a meal replacement may not be enough to help you gain weight. Instead, pair it with a balanced meal that includes protein, healthy fats, and carbohydrates.

In conclusion, almond butter and date smoothie is a delicious and healthy way to gain weight. With the right ingredients and some tips, you can make this smoothie more effective for weight gain and achieve your goals in a healthy way.

AVOCADO AND CHOCOLATE SMOOTHIE

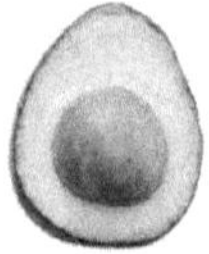

Avocado and Chocolate Smoothie is a delicious and nutritious beverage that is perfect for those who are looking to gain weight. Here is a step-by-step guide on how to make an avocado and chocolate smoothie that will help you gain weight.

INGREDIENTS:

1 ripe avocado

1 banana

1/2 cup unsweetened almond milk

1/2 cup plain Greek yogurt

1 tablespoon honey

2 tablespoons unsweetened cocoa powder

1/4 teaspoon vanilla extract

Ice cubes (optional)

INSTRUCTIONS:

Cut the avocado in half, remove the pit, and scoop the flesh into a blender.

Peel the banana and add it to the blender.

Pour the almond milk into the blender.

Add the Greek yogurt, honey, cocoa powder, and vanilla extract to the blender.

If you prefer your smoothie to be thicker, add a few ice cubes to the blender.

Blend all the ingredients together until smooth.

Pour the smoothie into a glass.

Garnish the smoothie with chocolate shavings or whipped cream if desired.

TIPS:

Choose a ripe avocado for the best flavor and texture. A ripe avocado should yield slightly to pressure when squeezed gently.

Use unsweetened almond milk to keep the smoothie low in sugar and calories.

Greek yogurt adds protein to the smoothie and helps to thicken it.

Use unsweetened cocoa powder to keep the smoothie low in sugar and calories.

Add honey for sweetness, but use it in moderation as it is still a form of sugar.

If you prefer a sweeter smoothie, add a few drops of liquid stevia instead of honey.

Use vanilla extract to enhance the flavor of the smoothie.

If you prefer your smoothie to be thicker, add more yogurt or avocado, or use less almond milk.

For an extra protein boost, add a scoop of protein powder to the smoothie.

Enjoy the smoothie as a meal replacement or as a post-workout snack to help you gain weight.

CHAPTER 5

PROTEIN-PACKED SMOOTHIES

GREEK YOGURT AND BERRY SMOOTHIE

Greek Yogurt and Berry Smoothie is a delicious and healthy way to gain weight. This smoothie is packed with protein, vitamins, and minerals, which makes it perfect for those who want to add some healthy calories to their diet. Here is a step-by-step guide on how to make a delicious Greek Yogurt and Berry Smoothie that will help you gain weight:

INGREDIENTS:

1 cup Greek yogurt

1 cup mixed berries (frozen or fresh)

1 banana

1/2 cup milk (any type of milk can be used, whole milk or almond milk works best)

1/4 cup honey

1/4 cup oats

1 tablespoon flaxseed oil (optional)

INSTRUCTIONS:

Start by adding the Greek yogurt to the blender. This will provide you with a good amount of protein, which is essential for weight gain.

Next, add the mixed berries to the blender. Berries are packed with vitamins and minerals, and they are also a good source of fiber.

Peel the banana and add it to the blender. Bananas are high in calories and potassium, which makes them a great addition to this smoothie.

Pour in the milk. Milk is a great source of calcium and vitamin D, which are essential for strong bones and teeth.

Add the honey. Honey is a natural sweetener that will give the smoothie a delicious taste.

Add the oats. Oats are a great source of complex carbohydrates, which will help to provide you with sustained energy throughout the day.

Finally, add the flaxseed oil. Flaxseed oil is high in healthy omega-3 fatty acids, which can help to reduce inflammation and promote heart health.

Blend everything together until smooth. You can add more milk if the smoothie is too thick.

TIPS:

Use frozen berries if you want a thicker smoothie. You can also add ice cubes to make it even thicker and colder.

If you don't like the taste of flaxseed oil, you can substitute it with coconut oil or any other healthy oil of your choice.

You can also add protein powder to the smoothie to increase the protein content.

If you are lactose intolerant, you can use lactose-free milk or a plant-based milk such as almond milk or soy milk.

If you want to add more calories to the smoothie, you can add nut butter such as almond butter or peanut butter.

Drink the smoothie immediately after blending to get the maximum benefits.

TOFU AND PEANUT BUTTER SMOOTHIE

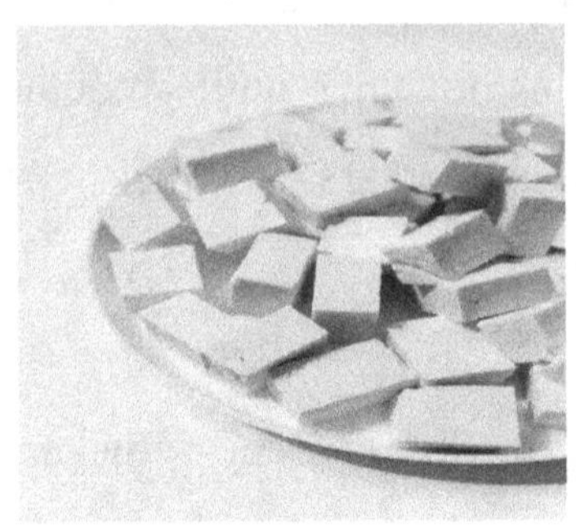

INGREDIENTS:

1 cup unsweetened soy milk

1/2 cup silken tofu

1/2 ripe banana

1 tablespoon natural peanut butter

1 tablespoon honey

1/2 teaspoon vanilla extract

1/2 cup ice cubes

INSTRUCTIONS:

In a blender, combine the soy milk, silken tofu, banana, peanut butter, honey, and vanilla extract.

Blend until smooth and creamy.

Add the ice cubes and blend again until smooth.

Pour the smoothie into a glass and enjoy!

TIPS:

Use unsweetened soy milk to keep the calorie count low.

Silken tofu is a great source of protein and will help to make the smoothie thicker and creamier.

Use a ripe banana for natural sweetness and added nutrition.

Natural peanut butter is a healthy source of fat and protein, but make sure to measure it out so you don't go overboard on calories.

Honey adds sweetness, but you can use a different sweetener like maple syrup if you prefer.

Vanilla extract adds flavor, but you can also add other flavorings like cinnamon or cocoa powder for variety.

Add more ice cubes for a thicker, frostier smoothie.

You can also add other ingredients like oats or chia seeds for extra nutrition and texture.

To increase the calorie count, you can use whole milk instead of soy milk or add more peanut butter or honey. Make sure to track your calorie intake and adjust the recipe accordingly to meet your weight gain goals.

CHICKPEA AND BANANA SMOOTHIE

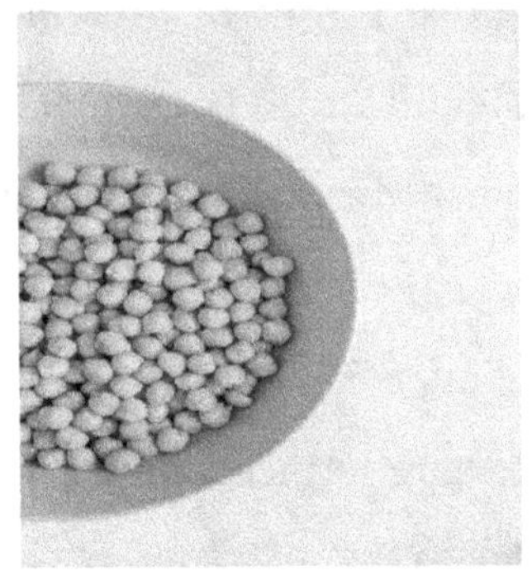

INGREDIENTS:

1 ripe banana

1/2 cup cooked chickpeas

1 cup unsweetened almond milk

1 tablespoon honey or maple syrup

1 teaspoon vanilla extract

1/2 teaspoon ground cinnamon

1/2 teaspoon ground ginger

1/4 teaspoon ground nutmeg

1 scoop vanilla protein powder (optional)

Ice cubes (optional)

INSTRUCTIONS:

Peel the banana and chop it into small pieces.

Drain and rinse the cooked chickpeas.

In a blender, add the banana, chickpeas, almond milk, honey or maple syrup, vanilla extract, cinnamon, ginger, nutmeg, and vanilla protein powder (if using).

Blend the ingredients until smooth and creamy.

If desired, add some ice cubes to the blender and blend again until the smoothie is cold and refreshing.

Taste the smoothie and adjust the sweetness and spice level according to your preference.

Pour the smoothie into a glass and enjoy immediately.

TIPS:

To make the smoothie even more nutrient-dense, you can add some spinach or kale to the blender. This will increase the fiber, vitamin, and mineral content of the smoothie without affecting its taste.

You can use any type of milk or milk alternative in this recipe. Almond milk, soy milk, coconut milk, or oat milk are all good options.

If you don't have a ripe banana, you can use frozen banana chunks instead. This will make the smoothie colder and thicker.

The protein powder is optional, but it can help you meet your daily protein needs if you're trying to gain weight or build muscle.

You can customize the spices in this recipe according to your taste. If you don't like cinnamon, you can use cardamom or cloves instead. If you like it spicy, you can add a pinch of cayenne pepper or black pepper.

To make the smoothie more filling and satisfying, you can add some nut butter, such as almond butter or peanut butter, to the blender. This will increase the healthy fats and protein content of the smoothie.

To make the smoothie more creamy and indulgent, you can add some coconut cream or Greek yogurt to the blender. This will make the smoothie thicker and richer.

QUINOA AND ALMOND MILK SMOOTHIE

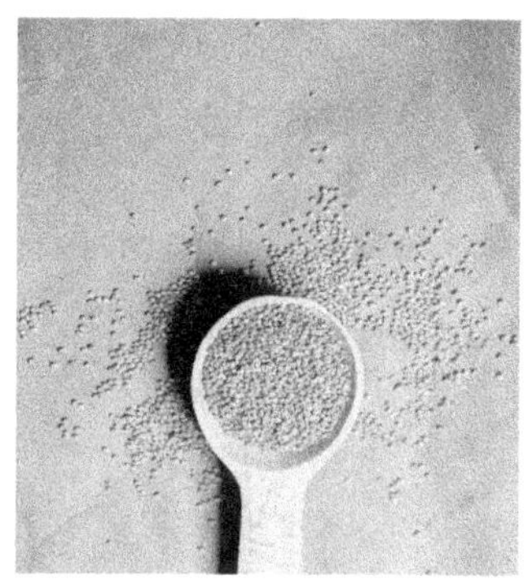

INGREDIENTS:

1/2 cup cooked quinoa

1 banana

1 cup unsweetened almond milk

1 tbsp almond butter

1 tbsp honey

1 tsp vanilla extract

1/2 tsp cinnamon

1/2 cup ice

INSTRUCTIONS:

Cook the quinoa according to package instructions and let it cool.

Add the cooked quinoa, banana, almond milk, almond butter, honey, vanilla extract, cinnamon, and ice to a blender.

Blend on high speed until smooth and creamy.

Pour into a glass and enjoy!

TIPS:

Use ripe bananas: The riper the banana, the sweeter it will be, which can help to balance out the nutty flavor of the quinoa and almond milk.

Use unsweetened almond milk: This will keep the sugar content of the smoothie low, while still providing a creamy and nutty flavor.

Add more protein: If you want to increase the protein content of the smoothie, you can add a scoop of your favorite protein powder or a tablespoon of chia seeds.

Use a high-speed blender: A high-speed blender will help to ensure that the quinoa is fully blended and doesn't leave any chunks in the smoothie.

Adjust the sweetness: Depending on your preference, you can add more or less honey to adjust the sweetness of the smoothie.

Serve immediately: This smoothie is best enjoyed immediately after blending, as the quinoa may become thick and grainy if left to sit for too long.

Overall, this Quinoa and Almond Milk Smoothie is a nutritious and filling option for weight gain, thanks to the protein and fiber in the quinoa and the healthy fats in the almond milk and almond butter. By following these tips, you can make a delicious and satisfying smoothie that will help you achieve your weight gain goals.

CHAPTER 6

SUPERFOOD SMOOTHIES

CHIA SEED AND BERRY SMOOTHIE

Chia Seed and Berry Smoothie is a delicious and healthy beverage that is perfect for weight gain. This smoothie is rich in nutrients, vitamins, and fiber, making it an ideal meal replacement for those who want to increase their calorie intake.

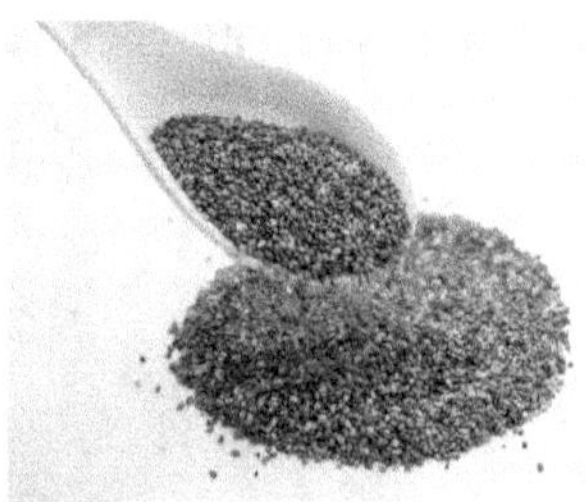

Here's a recipe for Chia Seed and Berry Smoothie for weight gain, along with some tips on how to make it even more effective:

INGREDIENTS:

2 tbsp chia seeds

1 cup mixed berries (fresh or frozen)

1 banana

1 cup milk (or dairy-free milk of your choice)

1 scoop protein powder (optional)

1-2 tbsp honey (optional)

INSTRUCTIONS:

Soak the chia seeds in water for about 5 minutes until they turn into a gel-like consistency.

Add the mixed berries, banana, milk, protein powder, and honey (if using) to a blender.

Blend the ingredients until smooth and creamy.

Pour the smoothie into a glass and sprinkle the chia seeds on top.

TIPS:

Add healthy fats: To increase the calorie content of your smoothie, you can add healthy fats such as avocado, nut butter, or coconut oil. These ingredients will also help keep you feeling fuller for longer.

Use a high-quality protein powder: Adding a scoop of protein powder to your smoothie will help increase your muscle mass and support weight gain. Look for a high-quality protein powder that contains all essential amino acids.

Choose your milk wisely: The type of milk you use can also impact the calorie content of your smoothie. Whole milk or a dairy-free alternative such as coconut or almond milk are good choices for weight gain.

Add extra fruit: If you want to increase the nutrient content of your smoothie, you can add extra fruit such as mango, pineapple, or kiwi. These fruits are high in fiber and antioxidants, which can support healthy digestion and immune function.

Experiment with different flavors: The beauty of making smoothies is that you can experiment with different flavors and ingredients. Try adding spinach, kale, or other leafy greens to your smoothie for an extra nutrient boost. You can also add spices like cinnamon, ginger, or turmeric for added flavor and health benefits.

Overall, Chia Seed and Berry Smoothie is a delicious and nutritious beverage that can help support weight gain when combined with a healthy diet and lifestyle. By following these tips, you can customize your smoothie to suit your taste preferences and nutritional needs.

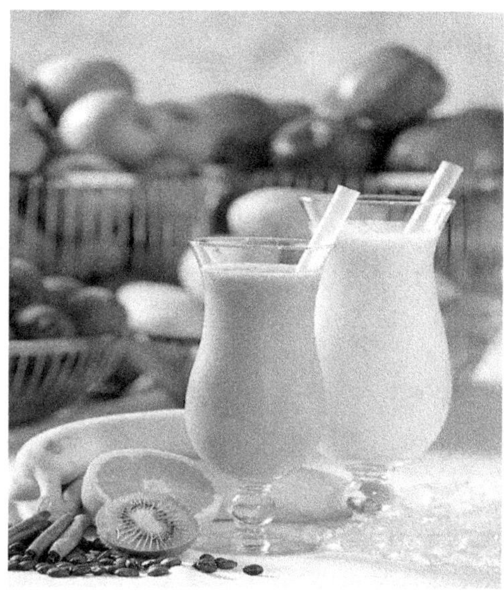

MATCHA AND BANANA SMOOTHIE

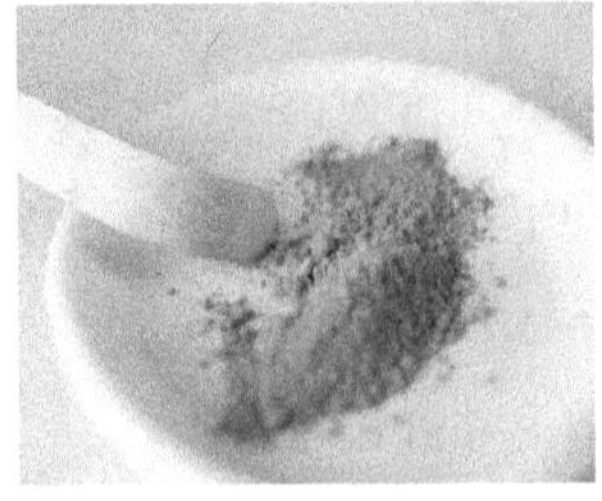 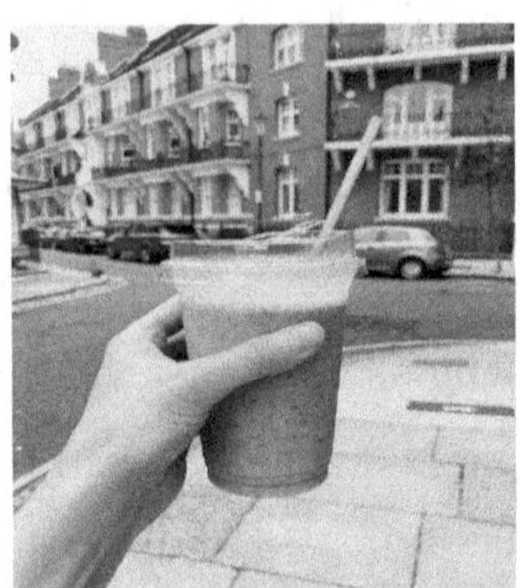

INGREDIENTS:

1 ripe banana

1 tsp matcha powder

1 cup almond milk (or milk of your choice)

1 scoop vanilla protein powder

1 tbsp honey

1 tbsp chia seeds

1 tbsp flax seeds

Handful of ice cubes

INSTRUCTIONS:

Start by peeling the banana and cutting it into smaller pieces.

Next, add the banana pieces into a blender.

Add 1 tsp of matcha powder to the blender.

Add 1 cup of almond milk (or milk of your choice) to the blender.

Add 1 scoop of vanilla protein powder. This will add some extra protein to your smoothie and help with weight gain.

Add 1 tbsp of honey. This will add some natural sweetness to your smoothie.

Add 1 tbsp of chia seeds. These are high in fiber and omega-3 fatty acids, which are both great for weight gain.

Add 1 tbsp of flax seeds. These are also high in fiber and omega-3 fatty acids.

Add a handful of ice cubes to the blender. This will help give your smoothie a nice, cold texture.

Blend all the ingredients together until smooth.

TIPS:

Use ripe bananas - they will add natural sweetness to your smoothie and be easier to blend.

Adjust the sweetness to your liking. If you prefer a sweeter smoothie, add more honey.

Use a high-quality matcha powder for best results.

Add extra milk or water if you prefer a thinner consistency.

If you have trouble digesting chia seeds, you can soak them in water for a few minutes before adding them to the blender.

If you don't have protein powder, you can leave it out.

To make this smoothie even more filling, you can add a scoop of peanut butter or almond butter.

Drink your smoothie as soon as possible after blending to get the most nutrients.

SPIRULINA AND MANGO SMOOTHIE

INGREDIENTS:

1 cup frozen mango chunks

1 banana

1 cup unsweetened almond milk

1 scoop spirulina powder

1 tablespoon honey (optional)

Ice cubes (optional)

INSTRUCTIONS:

First, gather all of the ingredients and have them ready on the countertop.

Add the frozen mango chunks and banana to the blender. Make sure to cut the banana into smaller pieces to make blending easier.

Pour in the unsweetened almond milk.

Add the spirulina powder to the blender. Spirulina powder is a great ingredient for weight gain because it is high in protein and other essential nutrients.

Add a tablespoon of honey if you prefer a sweeter smoothie. This is optional, so you can leave it out if you prefer.

Blend all the ingredients together until smooth. If the mixture is too thick, you can add some ice cubes to thin it out.

Once the smoothie is blended, pour it into a glass and enjoy!

TIPS:

If you want to increase the calorie content of the smoothie, you can add some nut butter like peanut butter or almond butter to the mix.

You can also add a scoop of protein powder to the smoothie to increase the protein content. This is especially helpful if you're trying to build muscle and gain weight.

Make sure to use unsweetened almond milk instead of sweetened almond milk to avoid adding unnecessary sugars to the smoothie.

Use frozen fruit instead of fresh fruit to make the smoothie thicker and creamier.

If you find the taste of spirulina too strong, you can start with a smaller amount and gradually increase it as you get used to the flavor.
You can also add other fruits like berries or peaches to the smoothie to change up the flavor.

Don't forget to clean your blender immediately after use to avoid any leftover residue.
I hope these tips help you create a delicious Spirulina and Mango smoothie that will aid in your weight gain journey!

MACA AND CHOCOLATE SMOOTHIE

INGREDIENTS:

1 banana, frozen

1 tbsp. maca powder

2 tbsp. cocoa powder

1 tbsp. honey

1 cup almond milk

1 scoop vanilla protein powder

1 cup ice

INSTRUCTIONS:

Begin by gathering all your ingredients and making sure they are all at room temperature.

Peel your frozen banana and chop it into small chunks.

Place the banana, maca powder, cocoa powder, honey, almond milk, vanilla protein powder, and ice into a blender.

Blend all the ingredients together for about 30-45 seconds, or until you get a smooth, creamy consistency.

Pour the smoothie into a glass and serve it immediately.

TIPS:

Use ripe bananas for a sweeter smoothie.

For a thicker consistency, use less almond milk and more ice.

Make sure to blend the smoothie well to ensure that all the ingredients are mixed together properly.

Adjust the sweetness of the smoothie to your liking by adding more or less honey.

You can use any type of milk you prefer in this recipe, such as soy, coconut, or cow's milk.

Use a high-quality vanilla protein powder to get the best flavor.

For an extra boost of nutrition, you can add some chia seeds, flax seeds, or hemp seeds to the smoothie.

To make the smoothie creamier, you can also add some Greek yogurt or avocado to it.

Don't forget to clean your blender immediately after use to prevent the smoothie from sticking to the blades.

Enjoy your delicious and healthy Maca and Chocolate Smoothie as part of a balanced diet and regular exercise routine to aid in weight gain!

CHAPTER 7

NUTRIENT-DENSE SMOOTHIES

SWEET POTATO AND PEANUT BUTTER SMOOTHIE

INGREDIENTS:

1 medium-sized sweet potato, peeled and cubed

2 tablespoons of peanut butter (or any nut butter of your choice)

1 cup of unsweetened almond milk (or any milk of your choice)

1 ripe banana

1 tablespoon of honey (optional)

1/2 teaspoon of cinnamon (optional)

1 scoop of vanilla protein powder (optional)

INSTRUCTIONS:

Preheat the oven to 375°F (190°C). Place the cubed sweet potato on a baking sheet and bake for 20-25 minutes, or until the sweet potato is soft and tender.

Once the sweet potato is cooked, let it cool down for a few minutes.

In a blender, combine the cooked sweet potato, peanut butter, almond milk, banana, honey, cinnamon, and vanilla protein powder (if using). Blend until smooth and creamy.

Taste the smoothie and adjust the sweetness as needed by adding more honey or banana.

Pour the smoothie into a glass and enjoy immediately.

TIPS:

To make this smoothie even creamier, you can add a tablespoon of Greek yogurt or coconut cream.

If you prefer a thicker smoothie, you can use frozen banana instead of fresh. Simply peel the banana, slice it, and freeze it overnight.

You can also add other ingredients to this smoothie to boost its nutritional value, such as chia seeds, flax seeds, or spinach.

If you don't have a blender, you can mash the cooked sweet potato and banana with a fork and mix in the other ingredients by hand.

This smoothie can be a great pre- or post-workout snack, as it provides a good balance of protein, carbohydrates, and healthy fats.

If you find that the smoothie is too thick or too thin, you can adjust the consistency by adding more or less almond milk.

This smoothie can be stored in the refrigerator for up to 24 hours, but it's best to consume it immediately to get the most nutritional benefits.

NUTRITIONAL VALUE OF SWEET POTATO

Sweet potatoes are a great source of nutrition and can be beneficial for weight gain. Here's an overview of the nutritional value of sweet potatoes:

Calories: A medium-sized sweet potato contains around 100-120 calories, which can be helpful for those trying to gain weight.

Carbohydrates: Sweet potatoes are a great source of complex carbohydrates, which provide sustained energy throughout the day. A medium-sized sweet potato contains around 25-30 grams of carbohydrates.

Fiber: Sweet potatoes are also high in fiber, which can aid in digestion and help you feel full for longer periods of time. A medium-sized sweet potato contains around 3-4 grams of fiber.

Protein: While sweet potatoes are not a significant source of protein, they do contain some amino acids that can be helpful for muscle building and repair.

Vitamins: Sweet potatoes are rich in vitamins A, C, and B6, all of which are important for overall health and immune function.

Minerals: Sweet potatoes are also a good source of potassium, which can help regulate blood pressure and support muscle function.

BROCCOLI AND PINEAPPLE SMOOTHIE

Broccoli and pineapple smoothie is a delicious and healthy drink that can help you gain weight if you consume it regularly. Here's how you can make it:

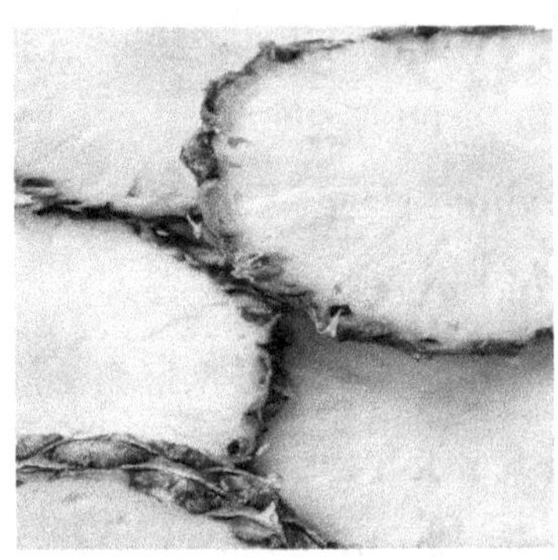
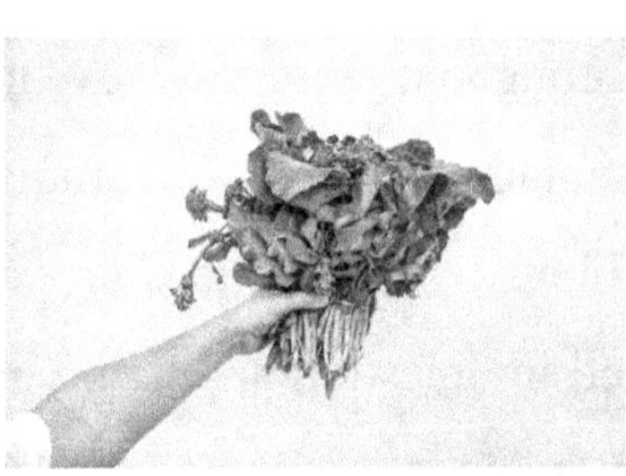

INGREDIENTS:

1 cup of broccoli florets

1 cup of frozen pineapple chunks

1 banana

1 cup of coconut milk

1 tablespoon of honey

1 teaspoon of vanilla extract

1 scoop of protein powder (optional)

INSTRUCTIONS:

First, rinse the broccoli florets thoroughly and cut them into small pieces.

Add the broccoli, frozen pineapple, banana, coconut milk, honey, and vanilla extract to a blender.

Blend all the ingredients until smooth and creamy.

Taste the smoothie and adjust the sweetness with more honey if necessary.

If you want to increase the protein content, add a scoop of protein powder to the blender and blend it again.

Pour the smoothie into a glass and serve it immediately.

TIPS:

Use frozen pineapple instead of fresh pineapple as it will make the smoothie more creamy and thick.

Use ripe bananas for a sweeter taste and a smoother texture.

If you're lactose intolerant, you can substitute coconut milk with almond milk or any other plant-based milk.

You can add more fruits or vegetables to the smoothie to increase its nutritional value.

To make the smoothie more filling, you can add a spoonful of peanut butter or almond butter.

Drink the smoothie immediately after blending as it may lose its nutritional value if left for too long.
You can also add some ice cubes to the blender to make the smoothie more refreshing.

To make the smoothie more enjoyable, you can garnish it with some chopped fruits, nuts, or shredded coconut.
By following these steps and tips, you can make a delicious and healthy broccoli and pineapple smoothie that can help you gain weight in a healthy way.

NUTRITIONAL VALUE OF BROCCOLI AND PINEAPPLE

BROCCOLI:

Broccoli is low in calories and high in fiber, making it an excellent food choice for weight gain. One cup of chopped broccoli (91g) contains:

31 calories

2.5g protein

6g carbohydrates

2.4g fiber

0.3g fat

135% of the recommended daily intake of vitamin C

116% of the recommended daily intake of vitamin K

11% of the recommended daily intake of vitamin A

6% of the recommended daily intake of iron

PINEAPPLE:

Pineapple is also low in calories and high in fiber, and it contains an enzyme called bromelain that can aid in digestion. One cup of diced pineapple (165g) contains:

82 calories

1g protein

21.7g carbohydrates

2.3g fiber

0.9g fat

131% of the recommended daily intake of vitamin C

76% of the recommended daily intake of manganese

10% of the recommended daily intake of vitamin B6

8% of the recommended daily intake of thiamin

How they help with weight gain:

Both broccoli and pineapple are low in calories but high in fiber, which can help you feel full and satiated for longer periods, reducing the chances of overeating and leading to weight gain.

Pineapple contains natural sugars that can help increase calorie intake and provide energy, which is essential for weight gain.

Broccoli is an excellent source of protein, iron, and other vitamins and minerals that are important for muscle growth and repair, which is necessary for weight gain.

Both broccoli and pineapple contain antioxidants and anti-inflammatory properties that can support overall health and help maintain a healthy weight.

Incorporating broccoli and pineapple into your diet, such as in a smoothie, can be a delicious and healthy way to help with weight gain. However, it's essential to remember that weight gain should be done in a healthy way by consuming a balanced and nutrient-dense diet and engaging in regular physical activity.

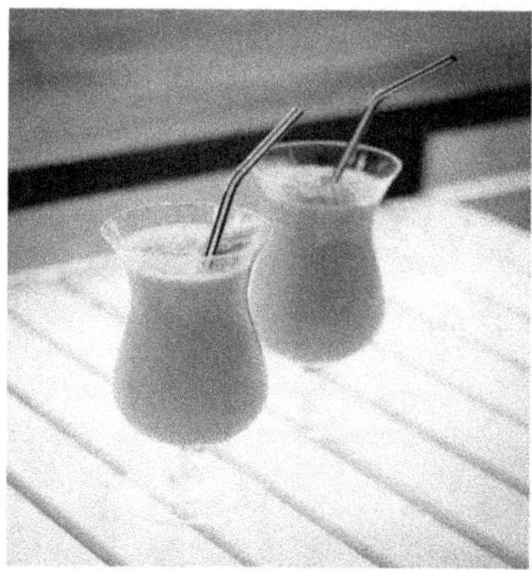

PUMPKIN AND CINNAMON SMOOTHIE

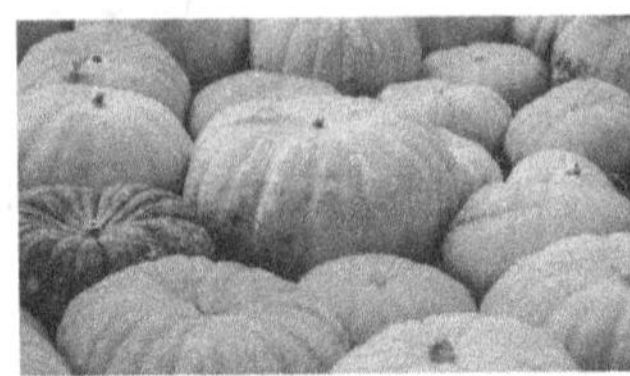 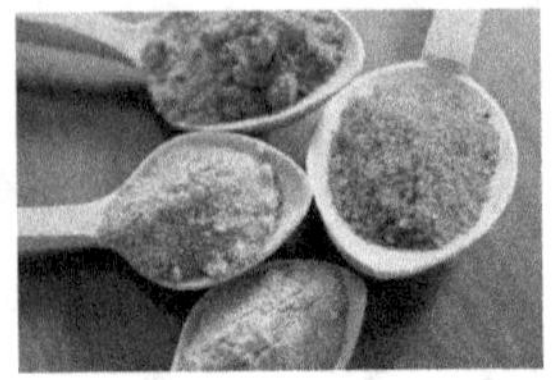

INGREDIENTS:

1 cup pumpkin puree

1 ripe banana

1/2 cup plain Greek yogurt

1/2 cup milk (you can use almond, soy, or cow's milk)

1/2 tsp cinnamon

1 tbsp honey

1/4 tsp vanilla extract

1/2 cup ice cubes

INSTRUCTIONS:

Add the pumpkin puree, banana, Greek yogurt, milk, cinnamon, honey, and vanilla extract to a blender.

Blend until smooth.

Add ice cubes and blend again until smooth.

Taste and adjust sweetness and consistency, if needed.

Serve and enjoy!

TIPS:

Use fresh or canned pumpkin puree. If using canned pumpkin puree, make sure it doesn't contain added sugar or spices.

Choose a ripe banana for sweetness and creaminess.

Greek yogurt adds protein and thickness to the smoothie, but you can use any other type of yogurt or skip it if you prefer.

Use your preferred type of milk, such as almond, soy, or cow's milk. Whole milk adds more calories and creaminess, but you can use low-fat milk or a plant-based alternative for a lighter version.

Cinnamon adds flavor and can also help regulate blood sugar levels.

Honey adds sweetness and can also provide some health benefits, but you can use other natural sweeteners such as maple syrup or dates.

Add ice cubes to make the smoothie colder and thicker, but you can skip them if you prefer a thinner consistency. Adjust the sweetness and consistency to your liking by adding more honey, milk, or ice cubes as needed.

You can also add other ingredients such as nut butter, protein powder, or chia seeds for extra nutrients and flavor.

Enjoy the smoothie as a snack or meal replacement, but make sure to balance it with other healthy foods and exercise to achieve a healthy weight gain.

NUTRITIONAL VALUE OF PUMPKIN AND CINNAMON AND HOW DOES IT HELP TO GAIN WEIGHT.

Both pumpkin and cinnamon have some nutritional value that can help with weight gain. Here's a brief overview of their nutrients and benefits:

PUMPKIN:

Low in calories but high in fiber: 1 cup of pumpkin puree contains only about 80 calories but provides 7 grams of fiber, which can help you feel fuller for longer and prevent overeating.

Rich in vitamins and minerals: Pumpkin is a good source of vitamin A, vitamin C, potassium, and iron, which are important for overall health and immune function.

Antioxidant properties: Pumpkin contains carotenoids, which are antioxidants that can protect against inflammation and cellular damage.

Cinnamon:

Low in calories but high in antioxidants: 1 teaspoon of cinnamon contains only about 6 calories but provides antioxidants that can protect against oxidative stress and chronic diseases.

Can help regulate blood sugar levels: Cinnamon has been shown to improve insulin sensitivity and lower blood sugar levels, which can reduce cravings and promote weight loss.

Anti-inflammatory properties: Cinnamon contains compounds that can reduce inflammation in the body, which is important for overall health and disease prevention.

In terms of weight gain, both pumpkin and cinnamon can provide some calories and nutrients that can support healthy weight gain when consumed as part of a balanced diet. Pumpkin is low in calories but high in fiber, which can promote satiety and prevent overeating. Cinnamon can help regulate blood sugar levels and reduce cravings, which can prevent overeating and weight gain. Additionally, adding these ingredients to smoothies or other dishes can provide flavor and variety to your diet, which can make it easier to maintain a healthy weight. However, it's important to consume these ingredients in moderation and balance them with other nutrient-dense foods to achieve a healthy weight gain.

ZUCCHINI AND BANANA SMOOTHIE

Zucchini and banana smoothie can be a healthy and delicious way to gain weight, as it is packed with vitamins, minerals, and healthy fats. Here is a recipe for a zucchini and banana smoothie that can help you gain weight:

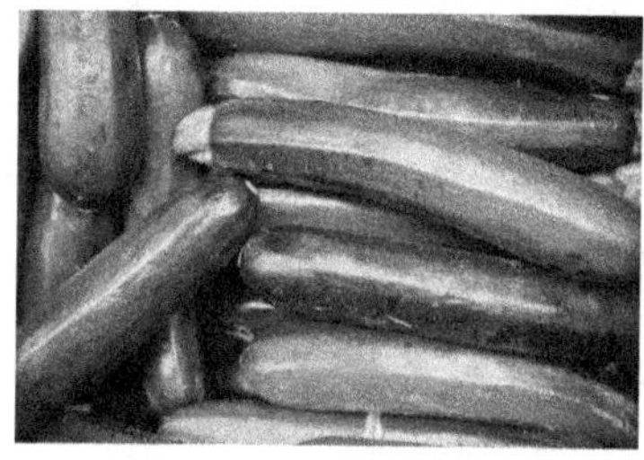

INGREDIENTS:

1 medium-sized zucchini, chopped

1 ripe banana, peeled and sliced

1/2 cup full-fat Greek yogurt

1/2 cup unsweetened almond milk

1 tablespoon honey

1 tablespoon chia seeds

1/4 teaspoon cinnamon

1/4 teaspoon vanilla extract

1/4 cup rolled oats

INSTRUCTIONS:

Wash and chop the zucchini into small pieces.

Peel and slice the banana.

Add the chopped zucchini, sliced banana, Greek yogurt, unsweetened almond milk, honey, chia seeds, cinnamon, vanilla extract, and rolled oats to a blender.

Blend on high speed until the mixture is smooth and creamy.

Pour the smoothie into a glass and enjoy!

TIPS:

Use a ripe banana: A ripe banana will add natural sweetness to the smoothie, making it more palatable. Plus, ripe bananas are easier to digest than unripe bananas.

Add healthy fats: To increase the calorie content of the smoothie, you can add a tablespoon of nut butter or coconut oil. This will also make the smoothie more filling and satisfying.

Use full-fat Greek yogurt: Full-fat Greek yogurt is rich in protein and healthy fats, which can help you gain weight. Plus, it will make the smoothie creamier and more delicious.

Use unsweetened almond milk: Almond milk is low in calories but high in nutrients. Using unsweetened almond milk will keep the calorie content of the smoothie low, while adding extra nutrients.

Add rolled oats: Rolled oats are a great source of complex carbohydrates, which can provide sustained energy and help you gain weight. Plus, they will make the smoothie more filling and satisfying.

Experiment with spices: Adding spices like cinnamon or nutmeg can enhance the flavor of the smoothie and make it more enjoyable to drink.

Drink the smoothie regularly: To see results, it's important to drink the smoothie regularly as part of a balanced diet and exercise program.

NUTRITIONAL VALUE OF ZUCCHINI

Zucchini is a low-calorie and nutrient-dense vegetable that is rich in various vitamins, minerals, and antioxidants. Here are the nutritional values for one cup (124 grams) of raw sliced zucchini:

Calories: 19

Protein: 1.4 grams

Fat: 0.3 grams

Carbohydrates: 3.5 grams

Fiber: 1.2 grams

Vitamin C: 32% of the Daily Value (DV)

Vitamin B6: 5% of the DV

Vitamin K: 8% of the DV

Folate: 6% of the DV

Potassium: 8% of the DV

Manganese: 8% of the DV

Magnesium: 6% of the DV

Zucchini also contains smaller amounts of other vitamins and minerals, such as vitamin A, vitamin E, thiamin, riboflavin, niacin, calcium, iron, phosphorus, and zinc.

In addition to its nutritional value, zucchini is also low in calories and carbohydrates, making it a great option for those who are watching their calorie intake or following a low-carb diet. Its high water and fiber content can also help promote feelings of fullness and aid in digestion.

CHAPTER 8

SMOOTHIES FOR BUILDING MUSCLE

WHEY PROTEIN AND BANANA SMOOTHIE

Making a whey protein and banana smoothie is a great way to help with weight gain, especially if you're an athlete or someone who engages in intense physical activity regularly. Here's how you can make a whey protein and banana smoothie for weight gain:

INGREDIENTS:

1 banana

1 scoop of whey protein powder

1 cup of milk (or almond milk)

1 tablespoon of honey

1 tablespoon of peanut butter

1/2 teaspoon of vanilla extract

1/2 teaspoon of cinnamon

5-6 ice cubes

INSTRUCTIONS:

Peel and slice the banana into small pieces and place them in a blender.

Add one scoop of whey protein powder to the blender.

Pour one cup of milk (or almond milk) into the blender.

Add one tablespoon of honey, one tablespoon of peanut butter, 1/2 teaspoon of vanilla extract, and 1/2 teaspoon of cinnamon to the blender.

Add 5-6 ice cubes to the blender.

Blend all the ingredients together until smooth.

Taste the smoothie and adjust the sweetness according to your preference by adding more honey if needed.

TIPS:

Use ripe bananas for a sweeter and creamier smoothie.

Use a high-quality whey protein powder for better results.

Use almond milk instead of regular milk for a dairy-free option.

Add more ice cubes if you prefer a thicker smoothie.

You can also add other ingredients such as oats, chia seeds, or flax seeds to increase the nutritional value of the smoothie.

Drink the smoothie within 30 minutes after making it to get the most benefit from the protein.

If you're trying to gain weight, drink this smoothie as a snack between meals or after a workout to increase your calorie intake.

If you're lactose intolerant, use a whey protein isolate instead of a concentrate, as it contains less lactose.

You can also use frozen banana slices instead of ice cubes for a thicker and creamier smoothie.

To make it more interesting, experiment with different fruit combinations and flavors, such as adding strawberries, blueberries, or raspberries.

NUTRITIONAL VALUE OF WHEY PROTEIN

Whey protein is a high-quality protein that is derived from milk. It is a complete protein, which means it contains all nine essential amino acids that your body cannot produce on its own. Here are some of the nutritional values of whey protein:

Protein: Whey protein is one of the most popular supplements among athletes and bodybuilders because it is a rich source of protein. A single scoop (30 grams) of whey protein powder contains approximately 25 grams of protein.

BCAAs: Branched-chain amino acids (BCAAs) are essential amino acids that help stimulate muscle protein synthesis. Whey protein is high in BCAAs, especially leucine, which is the most important amino acid for muscle growth and repair.

Low in fat: Whey protein is naturally low in fat, with most whey protein powders containing less than 1 gram of fat per serving.

Low in carbohydrates: Whey protein is also low in carbohydrates, making it an excellent protein source for people on low-carb diets.

High in calcium: Whey protein is a good source of calcium, which is important for maintaining strong bones and teeth.

High in immunoglobulins: Whey protein contains immunoglobulins, which are antibodies that help strengthen the immune system and protect against infections.

Digestion: Whey protein is easy to digest and absorb, making it an excellent choice for post-workout recovery or when you need a quick protein boost.

CREATINE AND BLUEBERRY SMOOTHIE

INGREDIENTS:

1 scoop of creatine powder

1 cup of frozen blueberries

1 banana

1 cup of almond milk (or milk of your choice)

1 tbsp of honey (optional)

1 tbsp of chia seeds (optional)

1 scoop of protein powder (optional)

INSTRUCTIONS:

Add 1 cup of frozen blueberries to your blender. Frozen blueberries are great because they add sweetness and thickness to the smoothie without adding any extra sugar.

Add 1 banana to the blender. Bananas are a great source of fiber, potassium, and natural sweetness.

Add 1 scoop of creatine powder to the blender. Creatine is a supplement that can help with muscle growth and strength, making it a great addition to a weight gain smoothie.

Add 1 cup of almond milk to the blender. You can use any milk of your choice, but almond milk is a great option because it's low in calories and high in nutrients like calcium and vitamin D.

If you want some extra sweetness, you can add 1 tbsp of honey to the blender.

If you want some extra nutrition, you can add 1 tbsp of chia seeds to the blender. Chia seeds are a great source of fiber, omega-3 fatty acids, and antioxidants.

If you want to increase the protein content of the smoothie, you can add 1 scoop of protein powder to the blender. Whey protein powder is a great option because it's high in protein and low in calories.

Once you've added all the ingredients to the blender, blend until smooth and creamy. Pour the smoothie into a glass and enjoy!

TIPS:

Use frozen fruit to make the smoothie thicker and creamier. If you don't have frozen fruit, you can use fresh fruit and add a handful of ice cubes to the blender.

Adjust the sweetness to your taste. If you prefer a sweeter smoothie, add more honey or use ripe bananas.

Use a high-quality blender to ensure that all the ingredients are blended thoroughly.

Drink the smoothie immediately after blending to get the most nutrients and freshness.

If you're trying to gain weight, make sure to eat a balanced diet and consume more calories than you burn. A weight gain smoothie can be a helpful addition to your diet, but it won't work if you're not eating enough overall.

NUTRITIONAL VALUE OF CREATINE AND BLUEBERRY

Creatine and blueberries are both nutritious and can provide various health benefits. Here are the nutritional values of creatine and blueberries:

CREATINE:

Creatine is a naturally occurring amino acid that is found in small amounts in animal products like meat and fish. It is also available in supplement form as creatine monohydrate. Here are the nutritional values of creatine:

Calories: 0

Protein: 0g

Carbohydrates: 0g

Fat: 0g

Creatine: 5g per serving (this may vary depending on the specific product)

Creatine is primarily used to increase muscle mass and strength, as it helps to regenerate ATP (adenosine triphosphate) in the body. It may also have other benefits, such as improving cognitive function, reducing inflammation, and protecting against certain neurological diseases.

BLUEBERRIES:

Blueberries are a type of fruit that are low in calories and high in nutrients. They are a good source of fiber, vitamin C, vitamin K, and antioxidants. Here are the nutritional values of 1 cup (148g) of raw blueberries:

Calories: 84

Protein: 1g

Carbohydrates: 21g

Fat: 0.5g

Fiber: 4g

Vitamin C: 24% of the Daily Value (DV)

Vitamin K: 36% of the DV

Antioxidants: Blueberries are rich in antioxidants, including anthocyanins, which give them their deep blue color. These antioxidants can help to protect the body against oxidative stress and inflammation.

Blueberries may have numerous health benefits, such as improving heart health, reducing inflammation, and supporting brain function. They are also a great choice for anyone looking to add more fruit to their diet without consuming too many calories.

BCAA AND MANGO SMOOTHIE

BCAA (branched-chain amino acid) and mango smoothie can be a delicious and nutritious drink to help with weight gain. Here's how to make it:

INGREDIENTS:

1 scoop of BCAA powder (unflavored or mango-flavored)

1 cup of frozen mango chunks

1 banana

1 cup of almond milk (or milk of your choice)

1 tablespoon of honey (optional)

Ice cubes (optional)

INSTRUCTIONS:

Put the frozen mango chunks, banana, BCAA powder, almond milk, and honey (if using) into a blender.

Blend all the ingredients until you get a smooth consistency.

If the mixture is too thick, add some ice cubes and blend again.

Pour the smoothie into a glass and enjoy!

TIPS:

Use a high-quality BCAA powder that is easily absorbed by your body.

Choose ripe and sweet mangoes to give the smoothie a natural sweetness.

Add more fruits like berries or pineapple to increase the fiber and nutrient content of the smoothie.

Consider adding a scoop of protein powder to further enhance the protein content of the smoothie.

You can also use coconut water instead of almond milk for a more tropical flavor.

Adjust the sweetness to your preference by adding more honey or using a different natural sweetener like maple syrup or stevia.

Drink the smoothie as a post-workout recovery drink or as a healthy snack in between meals to promote weight gain.

NUTRITIONAL VALUE OF BCAA AND MANGO

BCAA and mango are both nutrient-dense foods that offer a variety of health benefits. Here are the nutritional values of BCAA and mango:

BCAA:

Branched-chain amino acids (BCAAs) are essential amino acids that cannot be produced by the body and must be obtained through the diet or supplements. The three BCAAs are leucine, isoleucine, and valine.

Leucine:

5 calories per gram

2.5 grams per serving

Helps build and repair muscle tissue

Promotes protein synthesis and muscle growth

Isoleucine:

5 calories per gram

1.25 grams per serving

Helps regulate blood sugar levels

Supports energy production and endurance during exercise

Valine:

5 calories per gram

1.25 grams per serving

Supports muscle metabolism and growth

Helps prevent muscle breakdown during exercise

MANGO:

Mango is a tropical fruit that is rich in vitamins, minerals, and antioxidants.

99 calories per cup (165 grams)

1.4 grams of protein per cup

2.6 grams of fiber per cup

0.6 grams of fat per cup

100% of the daily recommended value (DRV) of vitamin C per cup

35% of the DRV of vitamin A per cup

20% of the DRV of folate per cup

8% of the DRV of potassium per cup

Mango is also a good source of other nutrients, including vitamin E, vitamin K, vitamin B6, and copper. Additionally, it contains beneficial plant compounds like polyphenols and carotenoids, which may have anti-inflammatory and antioxidant properties.

Combining BCAA and mango in a smoothie can provide a balanced blend of essential amino acids, vitamins, minerals, and antioxidants to support overall health and wellbeing.

HEMP PROTEIN AND CHOCOLATE SMOOTHIE

Hemp protein and chocolate smoothie is a delicious and healthy way to start your day or to have as a post-workout snack. Here's how to make it:

INGREDIENTS:

1 cup of unsweetened almond milk

1 banana

1 scoop of hemp protein powder

1 tablespoon of raw cacao powder

1 tablespoon of almond butter

1 teaspoon of vanilla extract

1 cup of ice

INSTRUCTIONS:

Start by adding the almond milk to your blender.

Peel the banana and add it to the blender.

Add the scoop of hemp protein powder, the raw cacao powder, and the almond butter.

Add the vanilla extract and the ice.

Blend everything until smooth and creamy.

If the smoothie is too thick, you can add more almond milk to thin it out.

Taste and adjust the sweetness if necessary. If you prefer a sweeter smoothie, you can add a few drops of liquid stevia or a teaspoon of honey.

Pour the smoothie into a glass and enjoy!

TIPS:

Use unsweetened almond milk to keep the smoothie low in calories and sugar.

Use ripe bananas for a sweeter taste and creamier texture.

Look for high-quality hemp protein powder that is organic and free of additives.

Raw cacao powder is high in antioxidants and adds a rich chocolate flavor to the smoothie.

Almond butter adds healthy fats and a nutty flavor to the smoothie.

Use a high-speed blender to blend everything smoothly and evenly.

If you're using frozen bananas, you may not need to add ice.

You can also add other ingredients to the smoothie, such as spinach, kale, berries, or chia seeds, for an extra boost of nutrients.

NUTRITIONAL VALUE OF HEMP PROTEIN AND CHOCOLATE

Hemp protein is a complete plant-based protein source, containing all nine essential amino acids, and is rich in fiber, iron, and healthy fats. Raw cacao powder is a good source of antioxidants and magnesium, which can support heart health and reduce stress. Together, they make a nutritious and delicious combination for a smoothie.

CHAPTER 9

SMOOTHIES FOR RECOVERY

TART CHERRY AND COCONUT WATER SMOOTHIE

Tart Cherry and Coconut Water Smoothie is a delicious and nutritious beverage that can help you gain weight. This smoothie is perfect for people who are trying to add some extra pounds to their body weight or for those who want to build muscle mass.

Here's how you can make a Tart Cherry and Coconut Water Smoothie for weight gain:

INGREDIENTS:

1 cup of frozen tart cherries

1 cup of unsweetened coconut water

1 scoop of vanilla protein powder

1 tablespoon of honey

1/2 banana (optional)

Ice cubes (optional)

INSTRUCTIONS:

Add the frozen tart cherries to a blender.

Pour the unsweetened coconut water into the blender.

Add a scoop of vanilla protein powder.

Add a tablespoon of honey to sweeten the smoothie.

If you want a creamier smoothie, add half a banana to the blender.

If you want your smoothie to be thicker and colder, add some ice cubes to the blender.

Blend all the ingredients until they are smooth and well combined.

Pour the smoothie into a glass and enjoy!

TIPS:

Use frozen tart cherries instead of fresh ones, as they will give your smoothie a thicker consistency.

Make sure to use unsweetened coconut water, as the added sugars in sweetened coconut water can negate the health benefits of the smoothie.

Choose a high-quality protein powder to ensure that you are getting all the essential amino acids that your body needs.

If you don't like the taste of honey, you can use other natural sweeteners like maple syrup or agave nectar.

To increase the calorie content of the smoothie, you can add a tablespoon of nut butter or some oats.

If you want to make the smoothie vegan-friendly, use a plant-based protein powder instead of whey protein powder.

Drink the smoothie after your workout, as it will help your muscles recover and grow.

Experiment with different ingredients to find the perfect combination for your taste buds.

NUTRITIONAL VALUE OF VALUE OF TART CHERRY AND COCONUT

Tart cherries and coconut are both nutrient-dense foods that offer a wide range of health benefits. Here's a breakdown of the nutritional value of each ingredient:

TART CHERRIES:

Tart cherries are a rich source of antioxidants and anti-inflammatory compounds that can help reduce the risk of chronic diseases. They are also a good source of fiber, vitamins, and minerals. A one-cup serving (140 grams) of frozen tart cherries contains:

Calories: 87

Carbohydrates: 22 grams

Fiber: 3 grams

Protein: 1.5 grams

Fat: 0.5 grams

Vitamin C: 10% of the daily value (DV)

Vitamin K: 7% of the DV

Potassium: 10% of the DV

Copper: 5% of the DV

Manganese: 14% of the DV

Coconut Water:

Coconut water is a refreshing and hydrating beverage that is naturally low in calories and rich in electrolytes, such as potassium and sodium. It is also a good source of vitamin C and magnesium. An 8-ounce (240-milliliter) serving of coconut water contains:

Calories: 45

Carbohydrates: 9 grams

Fiber: 3 grams

Protein: 1 gram

Fat: 0 grams

Vitamin C: 10% of the DV

Potassium: 17% of the DV

Sodium: 11% of the DV

Magnesium: 15% of the DV

Overall, tart cherries and coconut water can provide a variety of vitamins, minerals, antioxidants, and other beneficial compounds that can support overall health and wellbeing. Incorporating these ingredients into your diet in the form of a smoothie can be a great way to reap their nutritional benefits.

TURMERIC AND GINGER SMOOTHIE

Turmeric and ginger smoothie is a delicious and healthy drink that can help you gain weight. These two ingredients are known for their anti-inflammatory and antioxidant properties, and they can also aid in digestion and metabolism. Here's a recipe and some tips for making a tasty and nutritious turmeric and ginger smoothie:

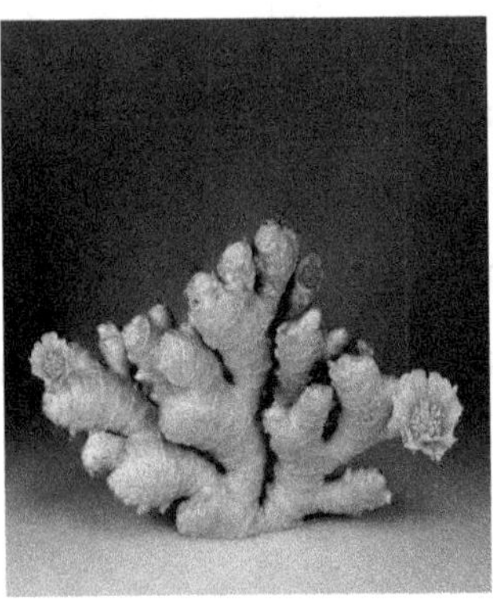
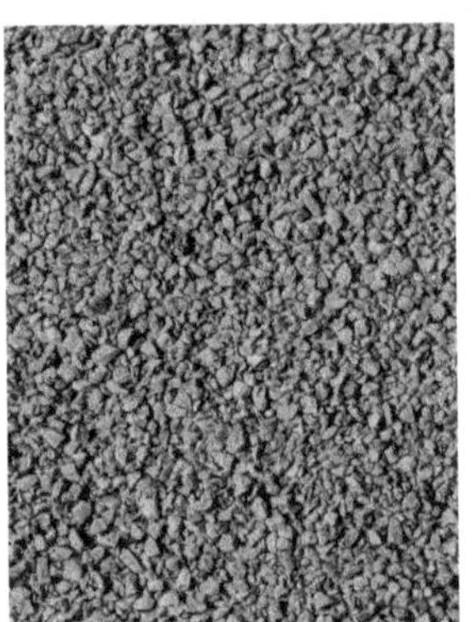

INGREDIENTS:

1 ripe banana

1 cup of unsweetened almond milk

1 tablespoon of grated fresh ginger

1 teaspoon of ground turmeric

1 tablespoon of honey or maple syrup (optional)

1/4 teaspoon of ground black pepper (optional)

INSTRUCTIONS:

Peel and slice the banana into small pieces.

Add the banana, almond milk, grated ginger, ground turmeric, and honey or maple syrup (if using) to a blender.

Blend on high speed until the mixture is smooth and creamy.

Taste the smoothie and add more honey or maple syrup if you prefer a sweeter taste.

Pour the smoothie into a glass and sprinkle the black pepper on top (if using).

Enjoy your delicious and healthy turmeric and ginger smoothie!

TIPS:

Use ripe bananas for a sweeter taste and creamier texture.

If you don't have fresh ginger, you can use ground ginger instead.

Add a scoop of protein powder to the smoothie to increase its protein content and help with weight gain.

Use a high-speed blender to ensure that the smoothie is smooth and creamy.

If you find the taste of turmeric too strong, start with a smaller amount and gradually increase it over time.

If you're using fresh turmeric instead of ground turmeric, be careful as it can stain your clothes and skin.

Black pepper can enhance the absorption of turmeric, so consider adding it to your smoothie.

Drink the smoothie immediately after making it to get the most nutrients from the ingredients.

PINEAPPLE AND CUCUMBER SMOOTHIE

Pineapple and cucumber smoothie is a delicious and healthy beverage that can be a great addition to your diet if you are looking to gain weight. Here's a recipe to help you make this smoothie:

INGREDIENTS:

1 cup fresh pineapple chunks

1 small cucumber, peeled and chopped

1/2 cup Greek yogurt

1/2 cup coconut milk

1 tbsp honey

1 tbsp chia seeds

INSTRUCTIONS:

Add the pineapple, cucumber, Greek yogurt, coconut milk, honey, and chia seeds to a blender.

Blend the ingredients until they are smooth and well combined.

Taste the smoothie and adjust the sweetness as desired by adding more honey.

Pour the smoothie into a tall glass and serve immediately.

TIPS:

To increase the calorie content of this smoothie, you can add a scoop of protein powder or a tablespoon of nut butter. This will also help to keep you full for longer.

Use ripe pineapple for maximum sweetness and flavor. You can also use frozen pineapple if fresh is not available.

Choose a full-fat Greek yogurt to add creaminess and extra calories to the smoothie.

If you don't have coconut milk, you can use almond milk, soy milk, or regular milk as a substitute.

To make the smoothie more filling, you can add a handful of spinach or kale to the blender. This will increase the nutrient content of the smoothie without affecting the taste.

You can make a large batch of this smoothie and store it in the fridge for up to 24 hours. Just give it a quick stir before drinking.

STRAWBERRY AND ALMOND MILK SMOOTHIE

INGREDIENTS:

1 cup frozen strawberries

1 ripe banana

1/2 cup almond milk

1/2 cup Greek yogurt

2 tablespoons almond butter

1 tablespoon honey

1 scoop protein powder (optional)

INSTRUCTIONS:

Begin by gathering all of the necessary ingredients and placing them on your kitchen counter.

Add the frozen strawberries, banana, almond milk, Greek yogurt, almond butter, honey, and protein powder (if using) to a blender.

Blend on high speed until the mixture is smooth and creamy. If the mixture is too thick, add more almond milk as needed.

Once the smoothie is blended to your desired consistency, pour it into a large glass or bottle.

Enjoy your Strawberry and Almond Milk Smoothie immediately, or store it in the refrigerator for up to 24 hours.

TIPS:

For an even creamier smoothie, use frozen banana slices instead of fresh.

If you prefer a sweeter smoothie, add more honey or a few dates to the mixture.

To increase the calorie count of your smoothie, add a tablespoon of coconut oil or nut butter.

You can also add in some greens such as spinach, kale, or avocado to increase the nutrient density of your smoothie.

Experiment with different flavors and ingredients to find the perfect combination for your taste preferences and dietary needs.

CHAPTER 10

SMOOTHIES FOR MEAL REPLACEMENT

CHOCOLATE AND PEANUT BUTTER MEAL REPLACEMENT SMOOTHIE

INGREDIENTS:

1 banana

1/4 cup of rolled oats

2 tbsp of peanut butter

1 tbsp of cocoa powder

1/2 cup of unsweetened almond milk

1 scoop of chocolate protein powder

1-2 cups of ice

INSTRUCTIONS:

Peel the banana and break it into chunks. Place the banana chunks into a blender.

Add the rolled oats, peanut butter, cocoa powder, unsweetened almond milk, and chocolate protein powder to the blender.

If you prefer a thicker smoothie, you can use frozen banana chunks instead of fresh bananas. This will also eliminate the need for ice cubes.

Start blending the ingredients together at low speed. Gradually increase the speed until the mixture is smooth and creamy.

Add the ice cubes to the blender and continue blending until they are fully incorporated.

If the smoothie is too thick, you can add more almond milk or water to thin it out to your desired consistency.

Once the smoothie is ready, pour it into a glass and enjoy!

This recipe is a great meal replacement option because it's high in protein, healthy fats, and complex carbohydrates. The banana provides natural sweetness and a good source of fiber, while the rolled oats add a hearty texture and more fiber. The peanut butter provides a good source of healthy fats and protein, and the cocoa powder adds a delicious chocolate flavor without any added sugar. The chocolate protein powder is an optional ingredient, but it can help boost the protein content of the smoothie, making it more filling and satisfying. You can also add other ingredients such as chia seeds, spinach, or honey, to customize the recipe to your liking.

BERRY AND GREEK YOGURT MEAL REPLACEMENT SMOOTHIE

INGREDIENTS:

1 cup of mixed frozen berries (such as strawberries, blueberries, raspberries, and blackberries): Frozen berries are a great addition to smoothies as they add natural sweetness, texture and are a good source of fiber and antioxidants.

1/2 cup of plain Greek yogurt: Greek yogurt is a high-protein, low-fat option that adds creaminess and tanginess to the smoothie. It also contains probiotics that can help with digestion and boost the immune system.

1 banana: Bananas add natural sweetness and creaminess to the smoothie. They are also a good source of potassium, which is important for muscle and nerve function.

1/4 cup of rolled oats: Oats are an excellent source of complex carbohydrates, fiber, and protein, which make them a great option for sustained energy throughout the day. They also help to thicken the smoothie.

1 tablespoon of honey (optional): Honey adds extra sweetness to the smoothie, but you can omit it if you prefer a less sweet taste.

1/2 cup of milk (or milk substitute): Milk or milk substitutes such as almond milk or oat milk are good options for adding creaminess to the smoothie. They are also a good source of calcium and vitamin D.

INSTRUCTIONS:

Gather all the ingredients and place them in a blender.

Blend the ingredients on high speed until smooth and creamy. If the smoothie is too thick, you can add more milk to achieve the desired consistency.

Taste the smoothie and adjust the sweetness by adding more honey if desired.

Pour the smoothie into a tall glass and enjoy immediately.

This Berry and Greek Yogurt Meal Replacement Smoothie is a perfect option for breakfast or lunch on the go. It is packed with nutrients and provides a balanced mix of carbohydrates, protein, and healthy fats to keep you feeling full and energized throughout the day. It's also very versatile, and you can switch up the fruit or milk to create different variations of the recipe.

VANILLA AND BANANA MEAL REPLACEMENT SMOOTHIE

INGREDIENTS:

1 banana, sliced

1 scoop vanilla protein powder

1 cup unsweetened almond milk

1/2 cup plain Greek yogurt

1 tsp honey (optional)

1/2 tsp vanilla extract

1 cup ice cubes

INSTRUCTIONS:

Gather all the ingredients and prepare your blender. Make sure your blender is clean and ready to use.

Peel and slice the banana and add it to the blender.

Add one scoop of vanilla protein powder to the blender. This will give your smoothie a boost of protein, which can help you feel full and satisfied.

Add one cup of unsweetened almond milk to the blender. Almond milk is a great dairy-free alternative to regular milk and it adds a nice nutty flavor to the smoothie.

Add half a cup of plain Greek yogurt to the blender. Greek yogurt is high in protein and adds a creamy texture to the smoothie.

If you want your smoothie to be a little sweeter, add one teaspoon of honey to the blender. This is optional, so skip this step if you prefer a less sweet smoothie.

Add half a teaspoon of vanilla extract to the blender. This gives the smoothie a delicious vanilla flavor.

Finally, add one cup of ice cubes to the blender. This will help make your smoothie cold and refreshing.

Blend all the ingredients together until smooth and creamy. You may need to stop the blender and scrape down the sides a few times to ensure everything is well mixed.

Once the smoothie is fully blended, pour it into a glass and enjoy!

You can customize this recipe by adding other ingredients like spinach or kale for added nutrition. You can also try using different flavors of protein powder or adding other fruits like strawberries or blueberries. The possibilities are endless!

GREEN MEAL REPLACEMENT SMOOTHIE

INGREDIENTS:

1-2 cups of leafy greens (spinach, kale, chard, etc.)

1-2 cups of frozen fruits (banana, berries, mango, etc.)

1-2 tbsp of nut butter (peanut butter, almond butter, cashew butter, etc.)

1-2 tbsp of honey or maple syrup

1 scoop of protein powder (whey, soy, or pea protein)

1-2 cups of liquid (water, milk, or non-dairy milk)

OPTIONAL ADD-INS:

1 tbsp of chia seeds or flaxseeds

1/2 cup of rolled oats

1 tbsp of coconut oil or MCT oil

1/2 avocado

INSTRUCTIONS:

Choose your greens: Pick your favorite leafy greens or mix and match them for a nutrient-rich base. Spinach and kale are popular choices because they are mild in flavor and high in vitamins and minerals.

Add the greens to the blender: Add 1-2 cups of leafy greens to your blender and pulse until they are finely chopped.

Add the frozen fruit: Add 1-2 cups of frozen fruits to the blender. Frozen fruits add a creamy texture and natural sweetness to the smoothie. Bananas, berries, and mango are all great options.

Add the nut butter: Add 1-2 tablespoons of your favorite nut butter to the blender. Nut butter is a great source of healthy fats, protein, and fiber. Peanut butter, almond butter, and cashew butter are all delicious choices.

Add the sweetener: Add 1-2 tablespoons of honey or maple syrup to the blender for added sweetness.

Add the protein powder: Add 1 scoop of protein powder to the blender. Protein powder is an essential ingredient for a meal replacement smoothie because it helps keep you full and supports muscle growth. Choose whey protein if you consume dairy, soy protein if you don't, or pea protein if you prefer a plant-based option.

Add the liquid: Pour in 1-2 cups of liquid to reach your desired consistency. Water, milk, and non-dairy milk are all great options. If you want a creamier smoothie, try using coconut milk or almond milk.

Optional add-ins: For extra nutrition and calories, you can add chia seeds, flaxseeds, rolled oats, coconut oil, or avocado. Chia seeds and flaxseeds are excellent sources of fiber and omega-3 fatty acids, while rolled oats add fiber and complex carbohydrates. Coconut oil and avocado provide healthy fats that can help you feel fuller for longer.

Blend everything until smooth and well combined: Blend all the ingredients until the smoothie is thick and creamy. If the mixture is too thick, add more liquid to thin it out.

Taste and adjust if needed: Taste the smoothie and adjust the sweetness or thickness if needed. If you want a sweeter smoothie, add more honey or maple syrup. If you want a thicker smoothie, add more frozen fruit or oats.

Pour into a glass or container and enjoy: Pour the smoothie into a glass or container and enjoy immediately. You can also store any leftovers in the fridge for up to 24 hours.

Green meal replacement smoothies are an excellent way to add more nutrients and calories to your diet. With the right combination of ingredients, you can create a smoothie that is not only delicious but also satisfying and filling. Experiment with different greens, fruits, and add-ins to find your perfect

CHAPTER 11

SMOOTHIES FOR SPECIFIC DIETARY NEEDS

GLUTEN-FREE SMOOTHIES

Making gluten-free smoothies is easy and can be done in a few simple steps. Here are some tips to help you make delicious and healthy gluten-free smoothies:

Choose gluten-free ingredients: Make sure that all the ingredients you use are gluten-free. This includes fresh or frozen fruits, vegetables, yogurt, milk, nut butter, honey, maple syrup, and other sweeteners.

Use gluten-free protein powder: If you want to add protein powder to your smoothie, make sure it's gluten-free. You can use whey protein isolate, pea protein, hemp protein, or other gluten-free options.

Avoid gluten-containing additives: Be careful with additives like malt, barley, and wheat germ, which contain gluten. Also, be careful with store-bought smoothie mixes, as they may contain gluten.

Use a blender that is easy to clean: To avoid cross-contamination, use a blender that is easy to clean or has removable blades that can be washed separately.

Experiment with different ingredients: There are plenty of gluten-free ingredients you can use to make delicious smoothies. Try using coconut milk, almond milk, or soy milk as a base, and experiment with different fruits and vegetables to find your favorite combinations.

Here's an example recipe for a gluten-free smoothie:

INGREDIENTS:

1 banana

1 cup frozen strawberries

1 cup unsweetened almond milk

1 scoop vanilla whey protein powder (or gluten-free protein powder of your choice)

1 tbsp honey (optional)

INSTRUCTIONS:

Add all the ingredients to a blender and blend until smooth.

If the smoothie is too thick, add more almond milk until you reach the desired consistency.

Pour the smoothie into a glass and enjoy!

DAIRY-FREE SMOOTHIES

Dairy-free smoothies are a great way to enjoy a healthy and delicious drink without using any animal products. Here are some tips on how to make dairy-free smoothies:

Choose a non-dairy milk: Instead of using cow's milk, choose a non-dairy milk such as almond milk, soy milk, coconut milk, oat milk, or rice milk. These milks are available at most grocery stores.

Use frozen fruit: Frozen fruit is perfect for making smoothies because it creates a thicker, creamier texture. Use frozen berries, mangoes, pineapples, bananas, or any other fruit of your choice.

Add a sweetener: If you like your smoothies sweet, you can add a natural sweetener like honey, maple syrup, or agave nectar. You can also use dates or stevia as a sweetener.

Add protein: To make your smoothie more filling, add some protein powder or a tablespoon of nut butter. This will also give your smoothie a creamy texture.

Add greens: If you want to make your smoothie more nutritious, add some greens like spinach, kale, or arugula. This will add some vitamins and minerals to your smoothie without affecting the taste.

Blend and enjoy: Once you have added all your ingredients, blend them together until smooth. Pour your smoothie into a glass and enjoy!

Here's a simple recipe for a dairy-free smoothie:

INGREDIENTS:

1 cup non-dairy milk (such as almond milk, soy milk, coconut milk, oat milk, or rice milk)

1 banana, frozen (or use fresh banana and add ice cubes)

1/2 cup frozen fruit (such as berries, mangoes, pineapples, or any other fruit of your choice)

1 tablespoon of natural sweetener (such as honey, maple syrup, agave nectar, or a few dates)

1 scoop protein powder (optional)

Handful of greens (such as spinach, kale, or arugula)

INSTRUCTIONS:

Gather all your ingredients and add them to the blender. Make sure the frozen fruit and banana are at the bottom of the blender so they blend up more easily.

Pour in the non-dairy milk of your choice. If you prefer a thicker smoothie, use less milk, and if you prefer a thinner smoothie, use more milk.

Add your natural sweetener to the blender. Honey, maple syrup, and agave nectar are popular choices. If you're using dates, make sure to remove the pits before blending.

Add a scoop of protein powder to your smoothie. This will give your smoothie an extra boost of protein and make it more filling. If you don't have protein powder, you can use a tablespoon of nut butter instead.

Add some greens to your smoothie. Spinach, kale, and arugula are great choices because they have a mild flavor that won't overpower the fruit. You can add as much or as little as you like.

Blend everything together until smooth. Start with a low speed and gradually increase the speed to make sure everything is well-blended. Stop the blender and scrape down the sides with a spatula if necessary.

Once your smoothie is well-blended, pour it into a glass and enjoy immediately. You can also top it with some additional fruit, nuts, or seeds for extra nutrition and texture.

That's it! Making a dairy-free smoothie is easy and customizable, so feel free to experiment with different fruits, sweeteners, and add-ins until you find the perfect combination for you.

VEGAN SMOOTHIES

INGREDIENTS:

1-2 cups of your favorite non-dairy milk (such as almond milk, coconut milk, or soy milk)

1-2 cups of your favorite frozen fruit (such as berries, mango, or pineapple)

1 ripe banana

1-2 tablespoons of sweetener (such as maple syrup, agave nectar, or honey substitute)

1 tablespoon of chia seeds or flaxseed (optional)

Ice cubes (optional)

INSTRUCTIONS:

Add the non-dairy milk to your blender.

Add the frozen fruit, banana, sweetener, and chia seeds or flaxseed (if using) to the blender.

Blend on high speed until smooth.

Add ice cubes (if using) and blend again until the smoothie reaches your desired consistency.

Pour the smoothie into a glass and enjoy!

You can also experiment with different combinations of non-dairy milk, frozen fruit, and sweeteners to create your own delicious vegan smoothie recipes.

LOW-SUGAR SMOOTHIES

Low-sugar smoothies can be a great way to enjoy the benefits of a delicious and healthy drink without consuming too much sugar. Here are some tips for making low-sugar smoothies:

Use low-sugar fruits: Instead of using high-sugar fruits like bananas, mangoes, or pineapples, try using low-sugar fruits like berries, apples, pears, or citrus fruits. These fruits are still sweet, but they contain less sugar.

Add vegetables: Vegetables can add nutrients and fiber to your smoothie while also helping to lower the overall sugar content. Try adding spinach, kale, cucumber, or celery to your smoothie.

Use unsweetened milk or yogurt: Many commercial brands of milk and yogurt contain added sugars. To keep your smoothie low in sugar, use unsweetened almond milk, coconut milk, or Greek yogurt.

Use natural sweeteners: If you still want your smoothie to be a bit sweeter, try using natural sweeteners like honey, maple syrup, or stevia. These options are lower in sugar than traditional sweeteners like sugar or agave nectar.

Limit the amount of fruit juice: Fruit juice can be high in sugar and can quickly add up in a smoothie. If you want to add juice to your smoothie, try using a small amount and diluting it with water.

Make your own smoothie blends: By making your own smoothie blends, you can control the ingredients and the amount of sugar. Try experimenting with different combinations of fruits and vegetables until you find a blend that you love.

CHAPTER 12

SMOOTHIES FOR BREAKFAST

BLUEBERRY AND OATMEAL SMOOTHIE

Blueberry and oatmeal smoothie is a delicious and nutritious breakfast option. Here's a simple recipe to make it:

INGREDIENTS:

1 cup blueberries (fresh or frozen)

1/2 cup rolled oats

1 banana

1 cup almond milk

1 tablespoon honey (optional)

1/2 teaspoon vanilla extract

ice cubes (optional)

INSTRUCTIONS:

Add blueberries, rolled oats, banana, almond milk, honey (if using), and vanilla extract to a blender.

Blend all the ingredients until smooth and creamy.

If you prefer a thicker smoothie, add a few ice cubes and blend again.

Pour the smoothie into a glass and serve immediately.

You can also add other ingredients to the smoothie, such as spinach, chia seeds, or protein powder, to increase its nutritional value. Enjoy your delicious and healthy blueberry and oatmeal smoothie for breakfast!

PEANUT BUTTER AND BANANA SMOOTHIE

Here is a simple recipe for making a delicious Peanut Butter and Banana Smoothie:

INGREDIENTS:

2 ripe bananas, sliced

1 cup unsweetened almond milk

2 tablespoons natural peanut butter

1 tablespoon honey or maple syrup

1/2 teaspoon vanilla extract

1 cup ice cubes

INSTRUCTIONS:

Add the sliced bananas, almond milk, peanut butter, honey or maple syrup, and vanilla extract to a blender.

Add the ice cubes to the blender.

Blend on high speed until the mixture is smooth and creamy.

If the mixture is too thick, you can add a little more almond milk or water to thin it out.

Pour the smoothie into glasses and serve immediately.

Optional: You can also add some protein powder or chia seeds to the smoothie for an extra boost of nutrition.

Enjoy your delicious and healthy Peanut Butter and Banana Smoothie for breakfast!

COFFEE AND CHOCOLATE SMOOTHIE

Here's a recipe for a Coffee and Chocolate Smoothie that you can enjoy for breakfast:

INGREDIENTS:

1 banana, frozen

1/2 cup brewed coffee, cooled

1/2 cup almond milk

1 tbsp cocoa powder

1 tbsp honey or maple syrup (optional)

1/2 tsp vanilla extract

1/2 cup ice cubes

INSTRUCTIONS:

Brew a cup of coffee and let it cool to room temperature.

Peel and slice the banana and place it in a blender.

Add the cooled coffee, almond milk, cocoa powder, honey or maple syrup (if using), vanilla extract, and ice cubes to the blender.

Blend on high until smooth and creamy.

Pour the smoothie into a glass and enjoy immediately.

You can also customize this recipe by adding protein powder or swapping out the almond milk for your preferred milk alternative. Enjoy your delicious Coffee and Chocolate Smoothie for a satisfying and energizing breakfast!

MANGO AND COCONUT SMOOTHIE

Here's a recipe for Mango and Coconut Smoothie that you can enjoy for breakfast:

INGREDIENTS:

1 ripe mango, peeled and chopped

1/2 cup coconut milk

1/2 cup plain Greek yogurt

1/2 cup ice cubes

1 tablespoon honey (optional)

Toasted coconut flakes for garnish (optional)

INSTRUCTIONS:

In a blender, add the chopped mango, coconut milk, Greek yogurt, ice cubes, and honey (if using).

Blend on high speed until smooth and creamy.

Taste and adjust sweetness, if needed, by adding more honey.

Pour the smoothie into a glass and garnish with toasted coconut flakes, if desired.

Serve immediately and enjoy your refreshing Mango and Coconut Smoothie for breakfast!

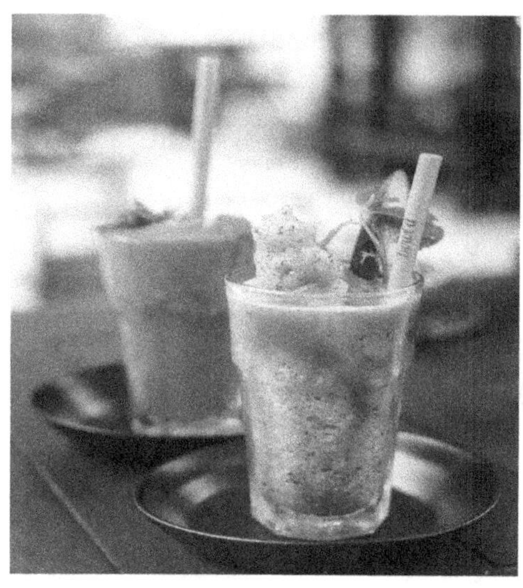

CHAPTER 13

SMOOTHIES FOR SNACKS

CINNAMON AND APPLE SMOOTHIE

INGREDIENTS:

1 medium apple, cored and chopped

1 banana, peeled and sliced

1 cup unsweetened almond milk

1/2 teaspoon ground cinnamon

1 tablespoon honey (optional)

1 cup ice cubes

INSTRUCTIONS:

Add the chopped apple, sliced banana, almond milk, ground cinnamon, and honey (if using) to a blender.

Blend on high speed until the mixture is smooth and creamy.

Add the ice cubes and blend again until the ice is completely crushed and the smoothie is thick and creamy.

Taste the smoothie and adjust the sweetness as needed by adding more honey.

Pour the smoothie into a glass and serve immediately.

Enjoy your delicious and healthy Cinnamon and Apple Smoothie for breakfast!

PEANUT BUTTER AND JELLY SMOOTHIE

Here's a simple recipe for a delicious Peanut Butter and Jelly Smoothie:

INGREDIENTS:

1 banana

1/2 cup frozen mixed berries

1/2 cup milk (or plant-based milk)

2 tablespoons peanut butter

1 tablespoon jelly or jam

1 tablespoon honey (optional)

Ice cubes (optional)

INSTRUCTIONS:

Peel the banana and break it into chunks. Put it in a blender.

Add the frozen mixed berries, milk, peanut butter, jelly, and honey (if using) to the blender.

Blend the ingredients until they are smooth and creamy.

If you want a thicker smoothie, you can add a few ice cubes to the blender and blend again.

Pour the smoothie into a glass and enjoy!

You can also garnish the smoothie with additional berries, chopped peanuts, or a drizzle of honey, if you like. Enjoy your delicious Peanut Butter and Jelly Smoothie for breakfast!

CHOCOLATE AND CHERRY SMOOTHIE

INGREDIENTS:

1 cup frozen cherries

1 banana

1/2 cup vanilla Greek yogurt

1/2 cup almond milk

1 tablespoon unsweetened cocoa powder

1/4 teaspoon vanilla extract

1-2 tablespoons honey (optional)

Ice cubes (optional)

INSTRUCTIONS:

Start by preparing the ingredients. Wash and pit the cherries, and peel the banana. You can also slice the banana into chunks to make it easier to blend.

In a blender, add the frozen cherries, banana, vanilla Greek yogurt, almond milk, unsweetened cocoa powder, vanilla extract, and honey (if using).

Blend the ingredients on high speed until smooth and creamy. If the mixture is too thick, you can add a few ice cubes and blend again until desired consistency is reached.

Check the taste and adjust the sweetness as needed by adding more honey or cocoa powder. Remember that the sweetness of the smoothie will depend on the ripeness of the fruit and your personal preference.

Once you're happy with the taste and consistency, pour the smoothie into glasses and serve immediately. You can also add a few slices of fresh cherries or a sprinkle of cocoa powder on top for extra flavor and presentation.

TIPS:

If you prefer a colder smoothie, you can use frozen banana instead of fresh banana, or add more ice cubes to the blender.

If you don't have almond milk, you can use any other type of milk or milk substitute, such as soy milk, oat milk, or coconut milk.

To make the smoothie vegan, you can use a non-dairy yogurt, such as coconut yogurt or soy yogurt, instead of Greek yogurt.

If you have a sweet tooth, you can also add a tablespoon of chocolate chips or a scoop of chocolate protein powder to the smoothie for extra indulgence.

Overall, this Chocolate and Cherry Smoothie is a delicious and healthy way to start your day or refuel after a workout. It's packed with antioxidants, fiber, protein, and healthy fats, and it's also gluten-free and low in calories. Give it a try and let us know how it turns out!

RASPBERRY AND ALMOND MILK SMOOTHIE

Here's a simple recipe for making a raspberry and almond milk smoothie:

INGREDIENTS:

1 cup frozen raspberries

1 banana, peeled and sliced

1 cup unsweetened almond milk

1 tablespoon honey (optional)

1/4 teaspoon vanilla extract (optional)

INSTRUCTIONS:

Add the frozen raspberries and sliced banana to a blender.

Pour in the unsweetened almond milk, honey (if using), and vanilla extract (if using).

Blend the ingredients until smooth, stopping to scrape down the sides of the blender if necessary.

Taste the smoothie and adjust the sweetness as desired by adding more honey.

Pour the smoothie into glasses and serve immediately.

Enjoy your refreshing raspberry and almond milk smoothie!

CHAPTER 14

SMOOTHIES FOR DESSERT

KEY LIME PIE SMOOTHIE

INGREDIENTS:

1 frozen banana

1/2 cup plain Greek yogurt

1/2 cup unsweetened vanilla almond milk

1/4 cup freshly squeezed key lime juice

1 tsp honey or agave nectar

1/2 tsp vanilla extract

1/4 tsp ground cinnamon

1/4 cup graham cracker crumbs

Ice cubes (optional)

INSTRUCTIONS:

Gather all the ingredients and have them ready for use. Ensure that the banana is frozen beforehand, as this will make the smoothie creamier and thicker.

Add the frozen banana, Greek yogurt, almond milk, key lime juice, honey or agave nectar, vanilla extract, and ground cinnamon to a blender.

Blend the mixture until it is smooth and creamy. If the the mixture is too thick, add a few ice cubes and blend again until it is at the desired consistency.
Once the smoothie is blended, pour it into a glass. You can choose to use a clear glass to show off the beautiful green color of the smoothie.

To garnish, sprinkle the graham cracker crumbs over the top of the smoothie. This will give it a nice crunch and add a bit of texture.
Serve immediately and enjoy your delicious Key Lime Pie Smoothie!

TIPS:
You can also add a few drops of green food coloring to enhance the green color of the smoothie if desired.
For a sweeter smoothie, you can adjust the amount of honey or agave nectar according to your taste preference.

If you don't have graham cracker crumbs, you can substitute them with crushed digestive biscuits or any other type of cookie you have on hand.

This recipe serves one, but it can easily be doubled or tripled to serve more people.

To make the smoothie even creamier, you can use full-fat Greek yogurt instead of plain Greek yogurt.

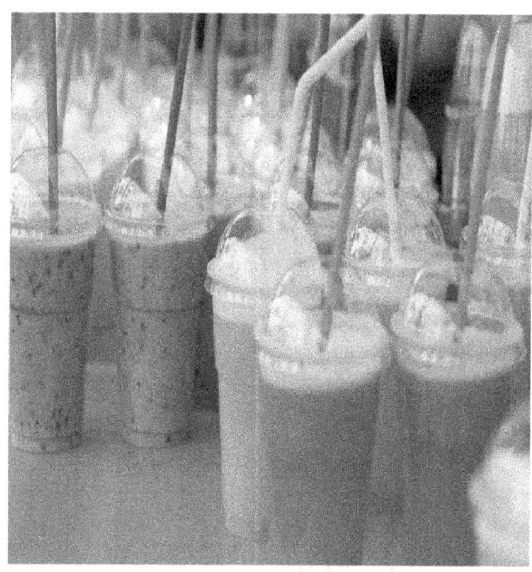

STRAWBERRY CHEESECAKE SMOOTHIE

Strawberry cheesecake smoothie is a delicious and easy-to-make smoothie that combines the flavors of strawberries and cheesecake. Here's a simple recipe to make this yummy smoothie:

INGREDIENTS:

1 cup fresh or frozen strawberries

1/2 cup plain Greek yogurt

1/2 cup milk (dairy or non-dairy)

1/4 cup cream cheese, softened

1 tbsp honey or agave syrup

1/2 tsp vanilla extract

1 cup ice cubes

INSTRUCTIONS:

Wash the strawberries and remove the stems. If you are using frozen strawberries, let them thaw for a few minutes before using them.

Add the strawberries, Greek yogurt, milk, cream cheese, honey or agave syrup, and vanilla extract to a blender. Blend the ingredients until they are smooth.

Add the ice cubes to the blender and blend again until the smoothie is thick and creamy.

Pour the smoothie into a tall glass.

If you want to give your smoothie the authentic taste of strawberry cheesecake, you can add some whipped cream and crushed graham crackers on top.

Serve and enjoy your delicious Strawberry Cheesecake Smoothie!

SOME VARIATIONS YOU CAN TRY:

You can use different types of berries, such as raspberries, blackberries, or blueberries, instead of strawberries to make a mixed berry cheesecake smoothie.

For a vegan version of this smoothie, use dairy-free yogurt and milk, such as soy milk or almond milk, and vegan cream cheese.

If you want to make your smoothie a little healthier, you can add some spinach or kale to the blender for some extra greens. It won't affect the taste of the smoothie and will add some nutritional value.

If you want to make your smoothie a little sweeter, you can add some more honey or agave syrup. Alternatively, you can add a banana to the blender for some natural sweetness.

You can also add some protein powder to the smoothie for an extra boost of protein. Just make sure to choose a flavor that compliments the taste of the smoothie.

BANANA BREAD SMOOTHIE

Banana bread smoothie is a delicious and healthy way to enjoy the flavors of banana bread in a drinkable form. Here's a simple recipe to make banana bread smoothie:

INGREDIENTS:

1 ripe banana

1/2 cup vanilla Greek yogurt

1/2 cup almond milk

1/4 cup rolled oats

1/4 tsp ground cinnamon

1/4 tsp ground nutmeg

1/4 tsp vanilla extract

1 tbsp honey

1 cup ice cubes

INSTRUCTIONS:

Peel the banana and cut it into chunks.

Add the banana, Greek yogurt, almond milk, rolled oats, cinnamon, nutmeg, vanilla extract, and honey into a blender.

Blend all the ingredients together until smooth and creamy.

Add the ice cubes to the blender and blend again until the ice is fully crushed and the smoothie is thick and frosty.

Taste the smoothie and adjust the sweetness as per your liking.

Pour the smoothie into a glass and serve immediately.

You can also add some chopped nuts or chocolate chips on top of the smoothie to give it an extra crunch and flavor. Enjoy your delicious and healthy banana bread smoothie!

MINT CHOCOLATE CHIP SMOOTHIE

Mint chocolate chip smoothies are a delicious and refreshing treat that can be enjoyed any time of day. Here's a simple recipe to make one:

INGREDIENTS:

1 banana, frozen

1 cup almond milk (or any milk of your choice)

1/2 tsp vanilla extract

1/2 tsp peppermint extract

2 tbsp chocolate chips

1 handful of spinach (optional)

1-2 tsp honey (optional)

ice cubes (optional)

INSTRUCTIONS:

Add the frozen banana, almond milk, vanilla extract, and peppermint extract to a blender.

If you like your smoothies a little thicker, add a handful of ice cubes to the blender.

Add the chocolate chips to the blender and blend everything together until smooth.

If you want to add a little extra nutrition to your smoothie, you can add a handful of spinach at this point. Blend again until smooth.

Taste the smoothie and adjust the sweetness to your liking by adding a little honey, if desired.

Pour the smoothie into a glass and enjoy!

Note: You can also garnish your mint chocolate chip smoothie with a few chocolate chips or a sprig of fresh mint for a little extra flair.

CHAPTER 15

SMOOTHIES FOR KIDS

BANANA AND NUTELLA SMOOTHIE

Banana and Nutella smoothie is a delicious and nutritious drink that kids are sure to love. Here's a simple recipe:

INGREDIENTS:

1 ripe banana

1 tablespoon Nutella

1/2 cup milk

1/2 cup ice cubes

Optional: honey or maple syrup for sweetness

INSTRUCTIONS:

Peel the banana and chop it into small pieces.

Add the banana pieces, Nutella, milk, and ice cubes to a blender.

Blend everything until smooth and creamy.

Taste the smoothie and add a little honey or maple syrup if you want it to be sweeter.

Pour the smoothie into a tall glass and serve immediately.

This recipe should make one large serving or two smaller servings. Enjoy!

STRAWBERRY AND VANILLA YOGURT SMOOTHIE

Here's a simple recipe for a Strawberry and Vanilla Yogurt Smoothie that kids will love:

INGREDIENTS:

1 cup frozen strawberries

1 cup vanilla yogurt

1/2 cup milk

1 tbsp honey (optional)

INSTRUCTIONS:

Prepare the ingredients. Rinse the frozen strawberries under running water to remove any ice crystals or debris. If you're using fresh strawberries, remove the stems and cut them into small pieces. Measure out the vanilla yogurt, milk, and honey and set them aside.

Add the ingredients to a blender. Place the frozen strawberries, vanilla yogurt, milk, and honey (if using) into a blender. Make sure the blender lid is tightly secured.

Blend the ingredients until smooth. Turn the blender on and blend the ingredients on high speed for about 30 seconds, or until the mixture is smooth and creamy. If the mixture is too thick, add a little more milk to thin it out.

Pour the smoothie into glasses. Once the mixture is blended to your desired consistency, turn off the blender and carefully remove the lid. Pour the smoothie into glasses and serve immediately.

Optional garnish. If you want to make the smoothie look more appealing to kids, you can add a few fresh strawberry slices on top of the smoothie, or sprinkle some chia seeds, granola, or coconut flakes on top for texture and flavor.

TIPS:

For a healthier version, you can substitute the vanilla yogurt with plain Greek yogurt and add a teaspoon of vanilla extract and a tablespoon of maple syrup for sweetness.

If you don't have a blender, you can use a food processor or an immersion blender to blend the ingredients.

To make the smoothie colder and more refreshing, you can add a few ice cubes to the blender before blending the ingredients.

If your kids have allergies or food intolerances, you can customize the recipe by using dairy-free yogurt or milk alternatives such as almond, soy, or oat milk.

ORANGE AND CARROT SMOOTHIE

Orange and carrot smoothie is a healthy and tasty drink for kids that is easy to make. Here's a simple recipe to make it:

INGREDIENTS:

2 medium-sized oranges, peeled and segmented

1 large carrot, peeled and chopped

1/2 cup of plain or vanilla yogurt

1/2 cup of ice cubes

1-2 tablespoons of honey (optional)

INSTRUCTIONS:

In a blender, add the peeled and segmented oranges, chopped carrot, yogurt, and ice cubes.

If you want to sweeten the smoothie, add 1-2 tablespoons of honey.

Blend all the ingredients together until the mixture becomes smooth and creamy.

Taste the smoothie and add more honey if needed.

Pour the smoothie into glasses and serve immediately.

You can also adjust the recipe to suit your child's taste by adding more or less yogurt or honey. Enjoy the delicious and healthy smoothie with your kids!

PEANUT BUTTER AND JELLY SMOOTHIE

Here's a simple recipe for making a delicious and healthy Peanut Butter and Jelly Smoothie that your kids will love:

INGREDIENTS:

1 cup of frozen strawberries

1 ripe banana

1/2 cup of creamy peanut butter

1/2 cup of milk (you can use almond or soy milk as a dairy-free alternative)

1 tablespoon of honey

1/2 teaspoon of vanilla extract

1/2 cup of ice cubes

INSTRUCTIONS:

Add the frozen strawberries, banana, peanut butter, milk, honey, and vanilla extract to a blender.

Blend the ingredients on high speed for about 30 seconds, or until the mixture is smooth and creamy.

Add the ice cubes to the blender and blend again for another 30 seconds, or until the ice cubes are crushed and the mixture is smooth and creamy.

Pour the smoothie into glasses and serve immediately.

Optional: You can garnish the smoothie with extra strawberries, peanut butter, or a drizzle of honey for added sweetness.

This recipe makes about 2 servings, so feel free to adjust the ingredients accordingly if you need more or less. Enjoy!

CHAPTER 16

SMOOTHIES FOR SPECIAL OCCASIONS

CHRISTMAS SMOOTHIE

Making a Christmas smoothie is a great way to add some holiday cheer to your morning routine. Here's a simple recipe to get you started:

INGREDIENTS:

1 cup of eggnog

1 banana

1/2 cup of frozen cranberries

1/4 tsp of ground nutmeg

1/4 tsp of ground cinnamon

1/2 cup of ice

INSTRUCTIONS:

Peel the banana and break it into pieces.

Add the banana, frozen cranberries, nutmeg, cinnamon, and ice to a blender.

Pour in the eggnog.

Blend on high speed until smooth and creamy.

If the smoothie is too thick, add a little more eggnog or water to thin it out.

Pour into glasses and enjoy your Christmas smoothie!

Optional: You can also add some whipped cream and a sprinkle of cinnamon on top for an extra festive touch.

HALLOWEEN SMOOTHIE

Halloween is a great time to get creative with your smoothie recipes and make something spooky and fun. Here's a recipe for a delicious and festive Halloween smoothie:

INGREDIENTS:

1 cup frozen mixed berries (you can use any combination of berries you like)

1 banana, peeled and sliced

1/2 cup vanilla yogurt (you can use plain or Greek yogurt as well)

1/2 cup milk (you can use any type of milk, such as almond, soy, or cow's milk)

1 tbsp honey (optional, for sweetness)

1 tsp vanilla extract (optional, for flavor)

2-3 drops of red food coloring (optional, for color)

2-3 drops of blue food coloring (optional, for color)

INSTRUCTIONS:

Gather all your ingredients and place them on your kitchen counter. Make sure your blender is clean and ready to use.

Add the frozen mixed berries, sliced banana, vanilla yogurt, milk, honey, and vanilla extract to the blender.

Blend the ingredients on high speed for 30-60 seconds or until the mixture is smooth and creamy. You can add more milk if the mixture is too thick.

Stop the blender and take a look at the color of your smoothie. If you want it to be more purple, add 2-3 drops of red food coloring and 2-3 drops of blue food coloring to the blender. If you prefer not to use food coloring, you can skip this step and enjoy the natural color of your smoothie.

Blend the mixture again for a few seconds until the food coloring is evenly distributed and the smoothie has turned a deep purple color.

Once the smoothie is ready, pour it into a glass and serve immediately. You can garnish it with whipped cream and Halloween-themed sprinkles or candy corn if you like.

Enjoy your spooky and delicious Halloween smoothie!

You can also experiment with different ingredients and flavors to create your own unique Halloween smoothie. For example, you can add pumpkin puree, cinnamon, and nutmeg for a pumpkin spice flavor, or use green food coloring and add spinach or kale for a monster-themed smoothie. Have fun and let your creativity run wild!

VALENTINE'S DAY SMOOTHIE

Valentine's Day Smoothie is a delicious and healthy way to show your love to your partner on this special day. Here's a simple recipe to make a Valentine's Day Smoothie:

INGREDIENTS:

1 cup frozen mixed berries

1 banana

1 cup unsweetened almond milk

1 tbsp honey or maple syrup

1/2 tsp vanilla extract

A pinch of cinnamon

INSTRUCTIONS:

Add the frozen mixed berries, banana, almond milk, honey/maple syrup, vanilla extract, and cinnamon to a blender.

Blend on high speed until the mixture is smooth and creamy.

Taste and adjust the sweetness if needed.

Pour the smoothie into two glasses and garnish with fresh berries, whipped cream or chocolate shavings, if desired.

Serve immediately and enjoy your Valentine's Day Smoothie with your loved one!

Note: You can also add some ice cubes to make the smoothie colder and thicker, or use other types of milk such as coconut or soy milk if you prefer.

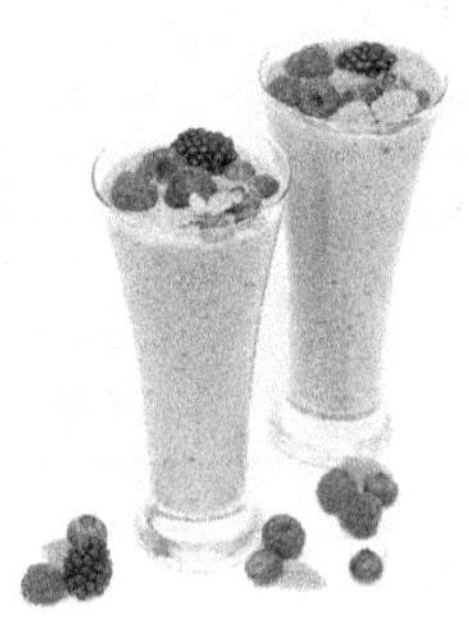

RECIPES TIMETABLE

Days	Recipes	Remark
1.		
2.		
3.		
4		

5		
6.		
7.		
8.		
9.		

10.		
11.		
12.		
13.		
14.		

15.		
16.		
17.		
18.		
18.		

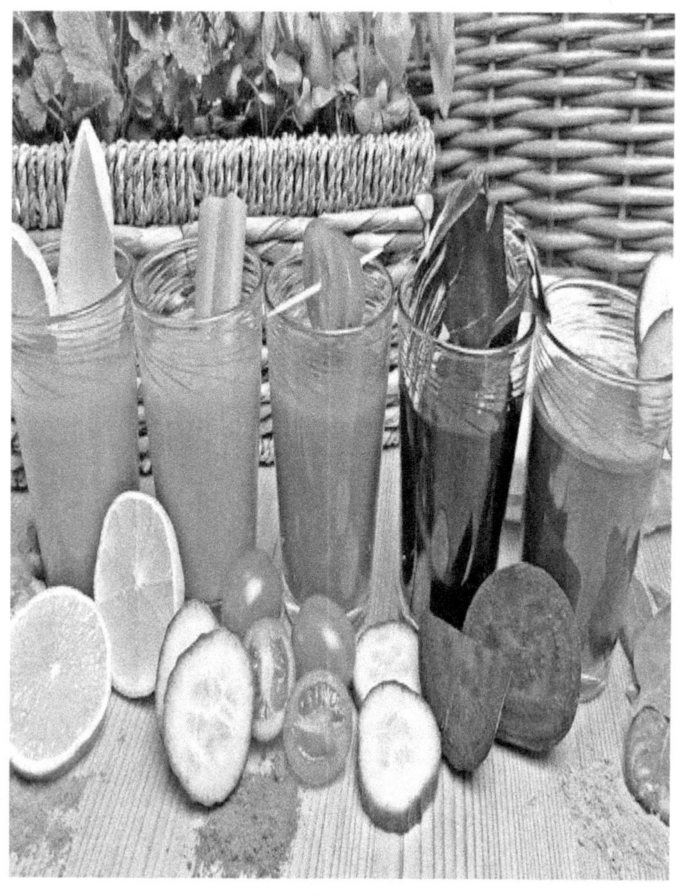